AF327901

REFLUX DISEASE

CAUSES, SYMPTOMS AND TREATMENT

DIGESTIVE DISEASES – RESEARCH AND CLINICAL DEVELOPMENTS

Additional books in this series can be found on Nova's website at:

https://www.novapublishers.com/catalog/index.php?cPath=23_29&series
p=Digestive+Diseases+-+Research+and+Clinical+Developments

Additional E-books in this series can be found on Nova's website at:

https://www.novapublishers.com/catalog/index.php?cPath=23_29&series
pe=Digestive+Diseases+-+Research+and+Clinical+Developments

REFLUX DISEASE

CAUSES, SYMPTOMS AND TREATMENT

GABRIELLA M. ESPOSITO
EDITOR

Nova Biomedical Books

New York

For permission to use material from this book please contact us:
Telephone 631-231-7269; Fax 631-231-8175
Web Site: http://www.novapublishers.com

NOTICE TO THE READER

LIBRARY OF CONGRESS CATALOGING-IN-PUBLICATION DATA

Reflux disease : causes, symptoms, and treatment / editor, Gabriella M. Esposito.
    p. ; cm.
  Includes bibliographical references and index.
  ISBN 978-1-61668-694-9 (hardcover)
  1. Gastroesophageal reflux. I. Esposito, Gabriella M.
  [DNLM: 1. Gastroesophageal Reflux--physiopathology. 2. Gastroesophageal Reflux--diagnosis. 3. Gastroesophageal Reflux--therapy. WI 250 R3318 2010]
  RC815.7.R387 2010
  616.3'24--dc22
                2010007617

ISBN: 978-1-61668-694-9

Published by Nova Science Publishers, Inc. ✝ New York

TABLE OF CONTENTS

PREFACE

Gastroesophageal reflux disease (GERD), or acid reflux disease is defined as chronic symptoms or mucosal damage produced by the abnormal reflux in the esophagus. This is commonly due to transient or permanent changes in the barrier between the esophagus and the stomach. This new book focuses on varied topics relating to reflux disease including: the role of mucosal inflammation in reflux disease, pharmacologic treatment of GERD, pediatric gastroesophageal reflux disease, paraesophageal hernias and laparoscopic antireflux procedures, minimally invasive treatments of gastroesophageal reflux disease, obstructive sleep apnea and GERD, and others.

Chapter I - Gastroesophageal reflux disease (GERD) affects up to one third of Western populations. It comprises three clinical entities: non erosive reflux disease (NERD), erosive esophagitis (ERD), and Barrett's esophagus (BE), the latter representing a premalignant lesion for the development of esophageal intraepithelial neoplasia and adenocarcinoma (EAC).

GERD is caused by recurrent exposure of esophageal mucosa to acidic and non-acidic refluxate. Contents are gastric acid, pepsin, bile acids and neutral peptidases released by pancreas and duodenum. Their interaction with squamous epithelium of the distal esophagus causes chronic inflammation (esophagitis), which is characterized by induction of inflammatory mediators like cytokines (IL-8, IL-1β), COX-2 and NFκB signaling pathway. Furthermore, GERD-associated esophagitis presents specific molecular and histological patterns that significantly differ from infection-associated mucosal inflammation.

Here we review the current knowledge about the expression of inflammatory mediators (cytokines, proteases, and reactive-oxygen species), mucosal infiltration of immune cell populations (Th1-, Th2-, and regulatory T cells) and signaling pathways (e.g. NFκB) related to GERD. We discuss further the potential use of inflammation-associated biomarkers for the assessment of GERD, the prediction of recurrence and the risk stratification for esophageal carcinogenesis.

Chapter II - Gastroesophageal reflux disease (GERD) affects women, men and children across worldwide demographic groups. The occurrence rate has increased over the past few decades, and epidemiological evidence suggests it will continue to do so into the foreseeable future. Left untreated, more serious diseases can result, including esophagitis and/or esophageal cancer. A number of treatment options are currently available for GERD, however the proton pump inhibitors (PPIs) are by far the most common treatment used. PPIs stop production of acid by shutting down the H^+/K^+-ATPase enzyme located in parietal cells. Evidence from recent studies suggests because PPI treatment is systemic, H^+/K^+-ATPase in tissues outside the stomach may also be impacted. These include the upper aerodigestive, otolaryngological, and esophageal regions. The use of PPIs may also be impacting H^+/K^+-ATPase within normally occurring human microbiota populations by raising pH levels, thereby potentially disturbing commensal bacteria and fungi. These colonies normally prevent opportunistic infections. Finally, there are two fundamentally different philosophical approaches chosen for PPI therapy by clinicians. The first pursues short-term treatment only when symptoms are present. The second treats continuously over time, which can lead to a number of undesired side effects. A further concern to clinicians is that while PPIs have been found to heal esophagitis, relapse occurs in the majority of patients shortly after discontinuing treatment. However, there are many negative implications for long-term use of PPIs, which also need to be considered. The impact on patient microbiota may be in ways not yet fully understood and therefore can complicate PPI therapy decisions and choices.

Chapter III - Gastroesophageal reflux disease (GERD) is one of the most common disorders in the pediatric population. Regurgitation of gastric contents into the lower esophagus is a physiologic event termed gastroesophageal reflux (GER) and cause minimal symptoms. However, when frequent symptoms impair quality of life and/or cause complications, it is called GERD. Symptoms can vary at different ages and can also affect other systems such as respiratory, dental and otolarygological organs.

Over the last decade, a more scientific and evidence-based understanding in this area has helped the professionals better understand GERD in children. In this chapter, we briefly discuss the advances in pathophysiology, epidemiology, clinical presentation, diagnostic modalities and management of pediatric GERD. Emerging data on natural history of Pediatric GERD are also reviewed.

Chapter IV - Paraesophageal hernia represents a rare acquired anatomical abnormality, comprising of migration of the stomach into the thoracic cavity and folding of the latter alongside the lower esophagus in a side-by-side manner. Due to the high complication rates of this condition, operative management is essential even in the absence of reflux symptomatology. Laparoscopic techniques provide the advantage of enhanced access to the mediastinum and precise dissection of the tissue surrounding the migrated stomach. Although the first reports on the outcome of laparoscopic fundoplication for the management of paraesophageal hernias exhibited good to excellent mid- and long term results with regard to symptom remission and reflux control, high recurrence rates led to skepticism on the efficacy and durability of primary suture hiatal closure. Hernia recurrence and intrathoracic wrap migration occurs in up to 42% of patients undergoing simple hiatoplasty due to either disruption of the diaphragmatic crura muscle fibers, wrap slippage through the intact hiatus or rupture of the sutures. Intrathoracic negative and intraabdominal positive pressures represent the most determinative physiological factors for these complications. The application of prosthetic material as reinforcement of the diaphragmatic defect in cases of paraesophageal hernia resulted in a dramatic decrease of recurrence rates and has an absolute indication in this patient population. However, mesh hiatoplasty is accompanied by several foreign-body complications, including mesh erosion, dysphagia, as well as severe epigastric pain. These complications result in a significant decrease of patients' quality of life and often require surgical reintervention. Therefore, mesh hiatoplasty should be applied in selected cases, with regard to the type and the size of the hiatal hernia, the surface of the hiatal defect and individual patient characteristics. Furthermore, clinical decisions should keep up with current evidence-based trends in order to minimize complications of antireflux procedures and improve patients' quality of life.

Chapter V - Karl Rokitansky first identified a relation between gastric acid and esophageal pathology in the 19th century [1]. While other physicians studied esophageal ulcerations, Asher Winkelstein was the first one to define reflux esophagitis in 1934. He documented a series of patients suffering from chronic substernal pain, heartburn, and regurgitation with diffuse esophageal inflammation on esophagoscopy. All patients in his series achieved some symptomatic relief with antacid therapy consisting of alkalinized intragastric milk [2]. Even decades after his original work, Winkelstein's initial description and findings of gastroesophageal reflux disease (GERD) remain largely unchanged.

Chapter VI - The normal physiology of the esophagus is complex and not completely understood. Recent evolution of diagnostic technology in the field of esophageal motility testing has helped the clinician in better understanding the normal physiology of the esophagus and in the management of patients with esophageal disorders. The purpose of this chapter is to give a comprehensive review of the normal anatomy of the esophagus with particular interest to its function, in light of the recent anatomic and physiologic findings obtained by high-resolution esophageal impedance manometry. The Authors describe the anatomic makeup of each area of the esophagus: the upper esophageal sphincter (UES), the body, and the lower esophageal sphincter (LES). Further emphasis is placed on the physiologic function of each anatomic area, and the mechanisms of the coordinated motor activity that ultimately results in the passage of food from the pharynx into the stomach.

Chapter VII- Gastroesophageal Reflux Disease (GERD) is a very common pathology in the general population and has been connected to various disorders of the respiratory tract for some time. At the otorhinolaryngological level, it has been considered a causal or favouring factor of chronic cough, laryngitis, sinusitis, laryngeal stenosis, and carcinoma of the larynx as well as respiratory trouble during sleep.

In: Reflux Disease: Causes, Symptoms and ...   ISBN: 978-1-61668-694-9
Editor: G. M. Esposito, pp. 1-36   © 2010 Nova Science Publishers, Inc.

Chapter I

THE ROLE OF MUCOSAL INFLAMMATION IN GASTROESOPHAGEAL REFLUX DISEASE

Arne Kandulski, Doerthe Kuester, Peter Malfertheiner and Thomas Wex[*]

Otto-von-Guericke University, Magdeburg, 39120 Magdeburg, Germany.

ABSTRACT

Gastroesophageal reflux disease (GERD) affects up to one third of Western populations. It comprises three clinical entities: non erosive reflux disease (NERD), erosive esophagitis (ERD), and Barrett's esophagus (BE), the latter representing a premalignant lesion for the development of esophageal intraepithelial neoplasia and adenocarcinoma (EAC).

GERD is caused by recurrent exposure of esophageal mucosa to acidic and non-acidic refluxate. Contents are gastric acid, pepsin, bile acids and neutral peptidases released by pancreas and duodenum. Their interaction with squamous epithelium of the distal esophagus causes

---

[*] Correspondence concerning this article should be addressed to: Dr. Thomas Wex, Ph.D. Department of Gastroenterology, Hepatology and Infectious Diseases, Otto-von-Guericke University, Magdeburg, Leipziger Str. 44, 39120 Magdeburg, Germany. Phone: (49)-391-6713106; Fax: (49)-391-6713105; E-mail: thomas.wex@med.ovgu.de.

chronic inflammation (esophagitis), which is characterized by induction of inflammatory mediators like cytokines (IL-8, IL-1β), COX-2 and NFκB signaling pathway. Furthermore, GERD-associated esophagitis presents specific molecular and histological patterns that significantly differ from infection-associated mucosal inflammation.

Here we review the current knowledge about the expression of inflammatory mediators (cytokines, proteases, and reactive-oxygen species), mucosal infiltration of immune cell populations (Th1-, Th2-, and regulatory T cells) and signaling pathways (e.g. NFκB) related to GERD. We discuss further the potential use of inflammation-associated biomarkers for the assessment of GERD, the prediction of recurrence and the risk stratification for esophageal carcinogenesis.

EPIDEMIOLOGY OF GERD-ASSOCIATED PATHOLOGIES

Gastroesophageal reflux disease (GERD) and its complications are still rising in incidence and prevalence, especially in Western countries [1,2]. About 20-30% of the adult population suffers from reflux-related symptoms such as heartburn and regurgitation. In the US 25 million patients complain about daily troublesome symptoms and the disease represents a burden for national health care systems [3]. Besides characteristic symptoms, many patients report about additional symptoms that are related to the esophagus adjacent organs (chronic cough, non-cardiac chest pain) or linked to functional disorders [4]. With the objective to define GERD as a spectrum of symptoms, the Montreal classification defines GERD as a disease caused by the refluxate of gastric contents into the esophagus that is associated with troublesome symptoms or complications [5]. GERD-related symptoms with or without complications were shown to lead to a burden of illness and loss of quality of life [6,7]. An association of dysphagia and GERD is considered as alarm symptom that needs further endoscopic evaluation in order to identify potential motility disorders, complications (strictures), malignancies or other diseases such as eosinophilic esophagitis [8].

Up to 60% of the patients do not present with endoscopic lesions in upper gastrointestinal endoscopy (non-erosive reflux disease, NERD), whereas 30% present with pathognomonic GERD-related erosive changes of the mucosa (erosive reflux disease, ERD) [9]. In about 5-10% of the patients, the esophageal squamous cell mucosa is replaced by a metaplastic columnar lined epithelium (Barrett´s esophagus, BE) that is considered as preneoplastic lesion for the development of distal esophageal adenocarcinoma (EAC) at an annual rate of 0.5-1% (Figure 1, [10-12]). Regarding health burden and affecting quality of life, there is no difference among the three entities of GERD [7,13].

Long-term studies showed that there is no progression of the different endoscopic manifestations of GERD from NERD to ERD or even to BE. Furthermore, even a regression of erosive lesion has been documented in up to 21% of the patients, which was explained by optimized acid suppressive therapies [14,15].

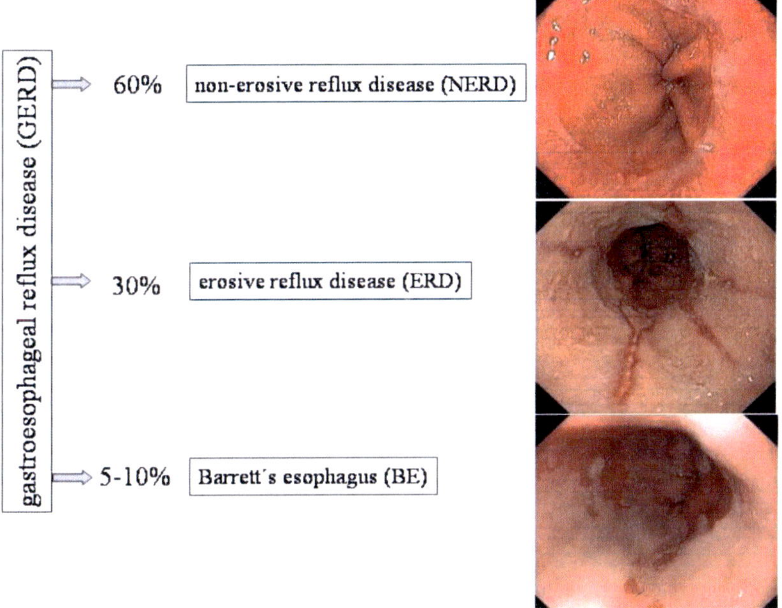

Figure 1. Endoscopic Manifestations of GERD.

Pathophysiology and Risk Factors for the Development of GERD

GERD is primarily caused by the pathological exposure of gastric or gastro-intestinal contents to the esophagus, but several other factors contribute to its multifactorial pathogenesis (Figure 2). The underlying pathomechanism is the transient relaxation of the lower esophageal sphincter (TLESR) that is associated with frequent episodes of reflux events to the distal esophagus [1,16,17]. The presence of a hiatal hernia, obesity and advanced age do not lead to GERD per se but impair the lower esophageal sphincter and are associated with more frequent reflux episodes [18,19]. Furthermore, medications interfering with smooth muscle cell function, such as nitrates, calcium channel blockers, theophylline or anticholinergics, lead to a reduced basale tone of the lower esophageal spincter (LES) and to more frequent TLESRs promoting GERD-related symptoms [20,21]. Many studies have been published about the interplay of *Helicobacter pylori* (*H. pylori)* and GERD with conflicting results [22]. The current concept does not relate the *H. pylori* infection to a higher incidence of GERD [23], however several studies have demonstrated a predominant pathophysiological role of *H. pylori* for chronic inflammation at the gastric cardia close to the squamocolumnar junction [24-26].

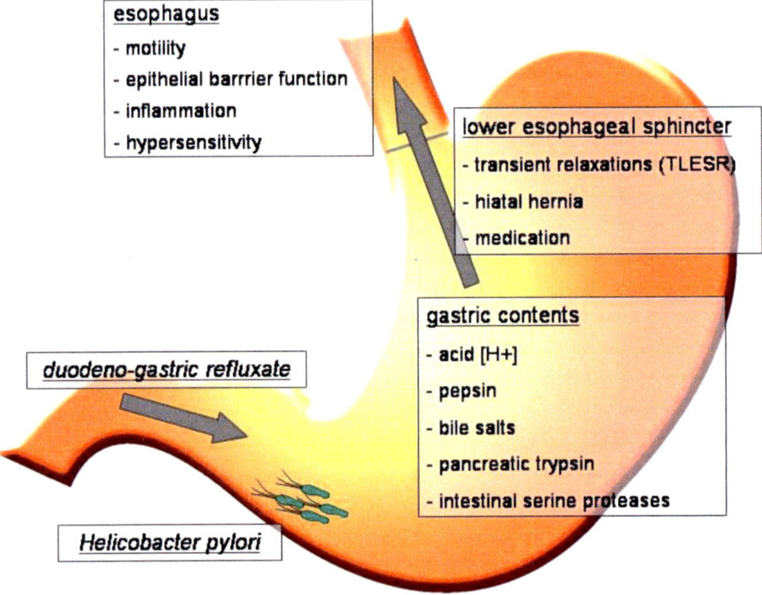

Figure 2. GERD – a multifactorial pathogenesis.

Heartburn and erosive esophagitis have been accepted as acid-induced symptoms or alterations for decades [27]. But a significant proportion of patients, especially with NERD, continue to have symptoms even when they are effectively treated with acid suppressive medication [28]. Furthermore, intraesophageal perfusion experiments showed an onset of heartburn appearing slower with higher pH but in 50% of the patients even at a pH of 6 [29].

Ambulatory pH monitoring showed that reflux episodes with pH between 4 and 7 were associated with symptoms in about 30% of the patients with GERD [30]. The application of combined pH and multichannel impedance monitoring (pH-MII) allows a detailed analysis of reflux events and provided evidence that even weakly acidic reflux episodes are sufficient to generate heartburn [31-33]. In addition to acid, reflux contains numerous other potential noxious contents, such as bile acids, pepsin, pancreatic trypsin or other gut-derived serine proteases. The action of these different agents under acidified conditions during reflux episodes may release (neuro-) inflammatory mediators (cytokines, neuropeptides, tryptase) from mucosal cell types (epithelial cells, inflammatory cells, mast cells). Furthermore it was demonstrated that these initial stimuli may be modified by central and peripheral (mucosal) mechanisms [34-37]. All together these processes lead to a persistent chronic inflammation of the esophageal mucosa that is considered as important risk factor in the pathogenesis of malignant diseases [38,39].

SPECIFIC HISTOMORPHOLOGICAL ALTERATIONS ASSOCIATED WITH GERD

The gastroesophageal junction (GEJ) represents histomorphologically a small but complex area, where stratified squamous epithelium of the distal esophagus "meets" columnar epithelium of the proximal stomach. Concerning the two main etiological causes, *H. pylori* and abnormal reflux, a gradient of histomorphological changes exists [40,41]. While both factors induce inflammation at the GEJ, only GERD is the pathophysiological determinant of esophagitis in the squamous epithelium of distal esophagus [40,42]. Abnormal exposure to gastric reflux, either acidic, minor acidic or alkali/ biliary-derived refluxate lead to infiltration of immune cells and specific histomorphological changes [41,42]. The most prominent histomorphological changes are the development of metaplastic columnar lined epithelium, representing either cardia-type mucosa or intestinal metaplasia (Barrett´s esophagus (BE)). The latter is associated with the development of intraepithelial neoplasia (formerly called dysplasia) and esophageal adenocarcinoma (EAC). Their molecular and histopathological alterations in esophageal carcinogenesis have been extensively reviewed by other groups [43-46]. Therefore, we will focus on the GERD-associated histomorphological alterations and inflammatory changes linked to esophagitis in patients having NERD, ERD and BE.

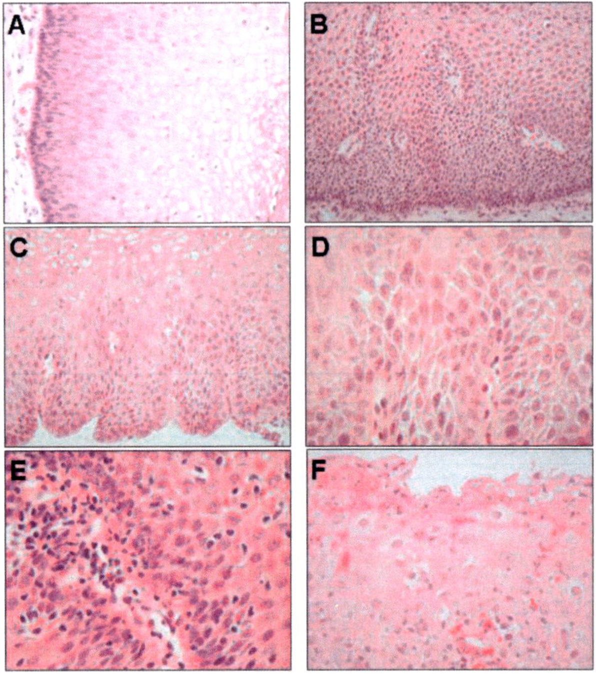

Figure 3. Histomorphological alterations of the esophageal mucosa associated with GERD. Compared to normal esophageal mucosa (A), in GERD, squamous epithelium demonstrates typical changes such as hyperplasia of basal cell layer (B), elongation and congestion of papillae (C), and spongiosis with dilatation of intercellular spaces (D). In NERD, infiltration of inflammatory cells is accentuated at the basal epithelial layers (E). Erosions with fibrinoid necroses infiltrated by cell debris and granulocytes are mainly observed in ERD (F).

At the first time, histopathological alterations were categorized by Ismail-Beigi in 1970. Besides mucosal inflammation; the presence of basal cell hyperplasia (BCH) and papillary elongation (PE) were described as GERD-specific changes (Figure 3) [47]. Hoopwood *et al.* identified a dilatation of intercellular spaces (DIS) of the esophageal mucosa of patients with GERD (Figure 3) [48], before Tobey *et al.* and others reintroduced this finding into the discussion of GERD [49,50]. These early studies were confirmed by various groups providing evidence that GERD-specific histological changes exist in general. The elongation of the papillae and basal cell hyperplasia were confirmed to present the most accurate histological parameters in the presence or absence of endoscopic criteria of GERD [41,51-53]. An impaired barrier function, which allows growth-promoting factors (e.g. salivary-derived EGF) penetrating into deeper layers of the esophageal mucosa and binding to its receptors on basal cells, was assumed to initiate repair processes and hyperplasia of basal cells [54]. The association of dilated intercellular spaces was confirmed by others [55,56] and nowadays the light microscopic analysis of DIS by the usage of hematoxilin & eosin and PAS staining adds an important additional feature to the histopathology in GERD [54,57]. Pathophysiologically, DIS is regarded as morphological correlate of impaired esophageal barrier function allowing toxic components of the refluxate to penetrate into esophageal mucosa initiating esophagitis and also perception of reflux-related symptoms [42]. In line with this model, dysregulation of tight junction components functionally linked to the regulation of epithelial permeability was described in animal models [58-60], whereas only one publications exist for humans so far [61]. In addition to DIS, other histological alterations such as interconnecting finger-like protrusions and cytoplasmic vacuoles have been described on subcellular level [62,63]. However, these alterations are only detectable by electron microscopy, and therefore have been investigated in few studies only, and are not applicable for routine histology.

With respect to the pattern of infiltrating immune cells, GERD-associated inflammation is characterized by a moderate infiltration of lymphocytes, macrophages and mast cells (Figure 3) [48,54,64]. The polymorphonuclear granulocytes defining the activity of inflammation are present in only 20-40% of patients with GERD [41,64-66]. Furthermore, an infiltration of eosinophils was identified in several patients with esophagitis that might be related to an overlap between eosinophilic esophagitis and GERD-associated inflammation. Therefore, an infiltration of eosinophils in GERD needs to be reevaluated critically [54,66]. However, it should be noted that the value of histology in diagnosing GERD is controversially discussed concerning its specificity in relation to this disease [41,54,67]. Potential reasons for these differences are the exact location of the biopsies and the use of PPIs in the in the inclusion criteria of different studies [54,58]. Recently, a scoring system for evaluating the histopathological alterations in relation to GERD was proposed [68]. Zentilin *et al.* analyzed basal cell hyperplasia, the elongation of papilla and dilatation of intercellular spaces to diagnose GERD histopathologically [68]. Whether the excellent interobserver agreement of >90% in this study can be achieved among pathologist in different countries needs still to be proven.

MUCOSAL CYTOKINE PATTERN IN GERD

Cytokine Pattern in the Esophageal Mucosa of Patients with GERD

In esophageal mucosa, the initial release of cytokines in response to infectious or chemical agents originates mainly from epithelial cells, and secondary from mucosa–resident immune cells. Among the early cytokines IL-8, RANTES, MCP-1 are released and stimulate the subsequent infiltration of immune cells, e.g. monocytes/macrophages, neutrophilic granulocytes, dendritic cells into the esophageal mucosa [37,69-73]. After infiltration, these cells become a significant cellular source for mucosal cytokines. The local concentration of these cytokines together with the presentation of luminal antigens are the major key factors for differentiation of distinct immune cells populations (Th1, Th2, Th17, Treg cells) that determine the activity, persistence and finally the resolution of inflammatory response (Figure 4). The final immune response is characterized by a local cytokine milieu expressed in the esophageal mucosa that can be regarded as "molecular pattern" of inflammation. Several studies were performed to describe these patterns in relation to the three entities of GERD. Applying array analysis, quantitative RT-PCR and protein-based methods (ELISA, immunohistochemistry) a Th1-dominating immune response was identified in patients with ERD and NERD. Besides various chemokines being upregulated [69-72], increased gene expression levels were identified for *IL-1α (69), IL-1β* [37,72,74,75], *IFN-γ* [72], *IL-18* [69]. For elevated *IL-8 and IL-1β* expression, a strong correlation with the extent of endoscopic lesions (ERD, Los Angeles classification) and histomorphological alterations was noted [37,69]. Generally, no differences were observed between ERD and NERD. Th1-related cytokines were similarly upregulated in both entities compared to reflux-negative controls.

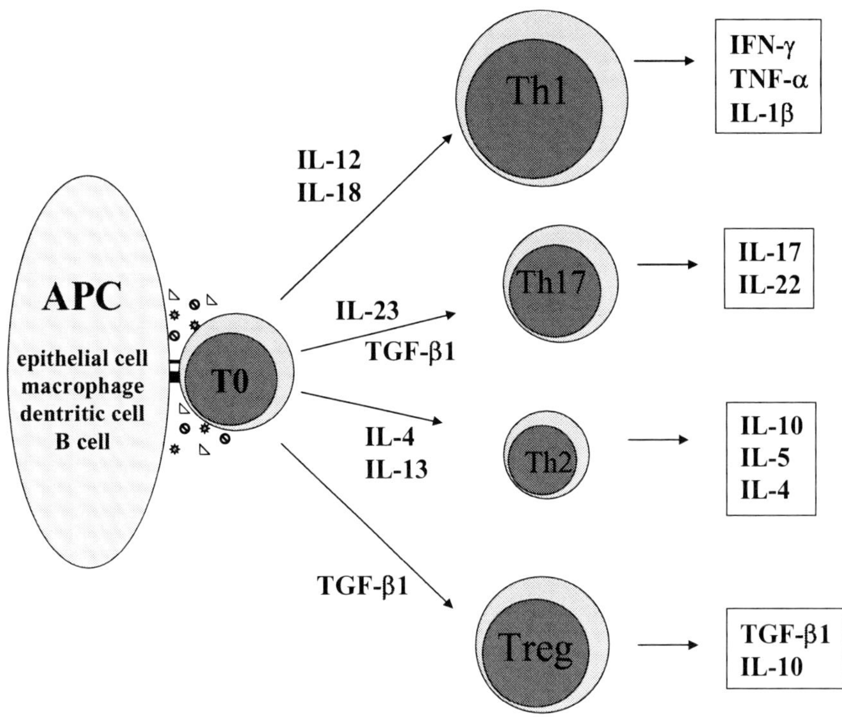

Figure 4. Immunological determinants of GERD-associated esophagitis. Luminal antigens are recognized by antigen-presenting cells (APC) that lead to the differentiation of different T cell lineages in the adaptive immune response. The various T cell lineages secrete different cytokines that further modulate the immune response that lead to different immunological characteristics of GERD-associated inflammation between ERD and BE.

For IL-8 being the best investigated cytokine in relation to GERD, the gene expression levels are always significantly induced in ERD and NERD compared to controls [37,70,76]). Some studies reported a stepwise increase of IL-8 levels from NERD to ERD [70]. The important role of IL-8 as chemokine is further supported by the fact that the esophageal mucosa expressed the corresponding receptors, CXCR-1 and –2, ubiquitously [77]. Interestingly, an upregulation of CXCR1 gene expression was solely determined in NERD [78], while both receptors remained unchanged in ERD [77]. As underlying mechanisms causing upregulation of IL-8 expression in relation to GERD, NFκB-signaling and Protease-activated receptor pathways were proposed. Isomoto *et al.* demonstrated an activation of NFκB immunohistochemically by the translocation of corresponding rel-subunits (p50 and p65) into the nuclei of IL-8-expressing cells in patients with ERD and NERD [79]. The fact that the initially elevated *IL-8 mRNA* levels normalized under acid suppressive therapy strongly suggests that acidic refluxate is the main culprit for IL-8 release [70]. Similar observation was made after surgical intervention. Successful Nissen fundoplication resulted in decreased *IL-8* mRNA levels in squamous epithelium and BE [80]. The response of cytokine expression to the effective antireflux therapy (either by medication or surgery) proves the causal role of the refluxate for inducing molecular and inflammatory changes in GERD. Furthermore, it is notable that elevated transcript levels of *IL-8, IL-1β and RANTES* in the esophageal mucosa were correlated to the recurrence of NERD implying that these molecules could be of potential use as predicative biomarkers [81].

IL-6 was identified as another important cytokine in GERD-related pathologies [82]. In children with GERD, esophageal biopsies obtained 2.3-fold more IL-6 than in controls, whereas systemic IL-6 and CRP levels were not altered [83]. In contrast to typical Th1-specific cytokines, IL-6 mediates diverse effects that can not solely categorized either to the Th1- or Th2 response [84]. Remarkably, this cytokine was associated with impaired cell-cell contacts (tight junctions, desmosomes) in a rat model [85] and motogenic activity of smooth muscle cells [82]. The important role of IL-6 for GERD was further supported by array analysis of microdisected esophageal epithelial cells from Wistar rats with esophagogastroduodenal anastomosis. Analyzing 207 out of 367 significantly altered genes, IL-6 signaling was identified as the most affected beside IL-2 and P38 MAPK pathways [86]. *In vitro* studies with the esophageal cell line Seg-1 demonstrated that low pH and bile aids induce IL-6 expression that lead subsequently to an activation of STAT3 pathway via Janus-kinase. This signaling cascade was suggested to induce of anti-apoptotic proteins such as Bcl-$_{XL}$ that mediate a higher resistance of esophageal epithelial cells to apoptosis [87]. This IL-6/STAT3 antiapoptotic pathway might be of importance for the prolonged survival of epithelial cells damaged by low pH and/or bile acids that develop dysplastic alterations and tumors. Based on these observations, a pathophysiological role of this molecule beyond the cytokine-mediated regulation of immune response can be assumed.

Between ERD and BE, Fitzgerald *et al.* identified significant differences in the immunological patterns between the two entities. The esophageal mucosa of patients with BE was characterized by rather low levels of proinflammatory (Th1-related) cytokines, whereas IL-4 (Th2-related) and IL-10 levels were abundantly expressed [72]. Furthermore, a gradient of cytokine expression was identified in these patients. Close to the new squamocolumnar junction, a significant induction of Th1-specific IL-1β and IL-8 levels was observed, distally the columnar lined mucosa of BE was associated with elevated IL-10 expression [88]. The predominant Th2-inflammatory response in BE was confirmed by Moons *et al.* who demonstrate a higher proportion of Th2-effector cells in BE compared to ERD, mainly higher numbers of plasma cells and mast cells in BE [89]. Interestingly, the numbers of IgE-secreting cells were higher in BE than ERD matching the increased IL-4 expression reported from others [72]. While IL-4 is known to initiate the development of intestinal metaplasia associated with mucin expression [90], the role of IL-10 is less defined. Historically, IL-10 and TGF-β1 were considered as major immunosuppressive cytokines that were balancing cell-mediated Th1-immune response. Nowadays, it has become clear that both molecules are key players for the differentiation and activity of regulatory T cells that control the activity of antigen-specific T cells (Figure 4, [91]). As of today, the role of these cells and their main cytokines (IL-10 and TGF-β1) has not been comprehensively studied in relation to GERD. Kandulski *et al.* studied the role of Treg cells at the cardia, and could not show an association of these cells or expression of both cytokines with GERD, but with the presence of *H. pylori* [92,93]. In children suffering from either eosinophilic esophagitis or GERD an increased number of FOXP3[+]CD25[+] were identified compared to healthy controls implying that Treg cells might be able to downregulate GERD-associated inflammation in the esophagus as well, but corresponding studies from adults are lacking [94].

FURTHER INFLAMMATORY MARKERS / PATHWAYS ASSOCIATED WITH GERD

Beside cytokines which are mainly studied in chronic inflammatory disorder, only a few other inflammatory pathways were studied in patients with GERD. Similar to other inflammatory diseases, COX-2 was found to be upregulated in GERD. Notably, patients with BE revealed higher immunohistochemically determined expression scores than those with ERD/NERD [95]. The regulation of COX-2 expression in BE by bile acids was studied *in vitro* using immortalized cell lines. Unconjugated bile acids induced CREB and AP-1-dependent COX-2 expression in Barrett's esophagus through activation of PI3K/AKT and ERK1/2 mediated by reactive oxygen species (ROS). Scavangers of ROS inhibited the induction of COX-2 implying a central role of ROS for involved pathways [96]. Vallböhmer *et al.* identified a stepwise increase of *Cox-2* transcript levels in the esophageal mucosa within the control – GERD – BE – intraepithelial neoplasia – adenocarcinoma sequence [97]. After Nissen fundoplication, the increased COX-2 expression of patients with GERD returned to levels similar to those observed in reflux-negative controls [98].

Another important regulator of chronic inflammation and carcinogenesis is the NFκB-signaling pathway that has been mainly studied in the context of distal adenocarcinoma which is the most complicated disease of BE. While, expression of NFκB-components (Rel-proteins, IκB-inhibitors) is not or only minimally detectable in normal healthy esophageal mucosa, its activation was gradiently increased in patients with GERD, BE and EAC with the latter showing highest induction of this pathway [99,100]. Notably, the activation of NFκB correlated inversely with the response to chemoradiotherapy in EAC [101]. Furthermore, the induction of NFκB-signaling in patients with EAC was associated with high expression levels of IL-8 and IL-1β [99,100]. *In vitro* studies with esophageal cell lines such as HET-1A supported the central role of NFκB-signaling in GERD. Acified medium (pH 4.5) induced NFκB activity that led subsequently to release of IL-6 and IL-8, two major cytokines in GERD. MAPK and PKC signaling pathways were identified as downstream regulatory pathways in the acid-mediated IL-6 and IL-8 expression via NFκB [102].

Taken into consideration that the gastroduodenal refluxate contains bile acids, Capello *et al.* studied the role of the bile acid Farnesoid X receptor (FXR) and bile-metabolizing genes. The upregulation of FXR, ilial bile binding protein, small heterodimer partner and the chemokines IL-8 and MIP-3α in the esophageal mucosa of patients with BE as well as their induction in an *in vitro* model (TE7 cells) by deoxycholic acid supports a pathophysiological role of these genes in patients exposed to duodenal-biliary refluxate [103].

ROS have been linked to chronic inflammatory disorders in various tissues [104]. Cheng *et al.* studied human esophageal lower esophageal sphincter (LES) circular muscle specimens and showed that the reduced tonus was restored after treatment with catalase, a scavenger of ROS. In contrast, incubation of LES-derived smooth muscle tissue from controls with H_2O_2 induced the release of platelet activating factor (PAF), prostaglandin E2 (PGE_2), and F2-isoprostane that were capable to reduce LES tone in human esophagitis [83]. Another study identified slightly increased levels of ROS in the esophageal mucosa of children with mild and moderate esophagitis, and concluded that ROS are in particular important for the initiation of severe GERD [105]. In line with this hypothesis other groups demonstrated a predominant role of ROS in the development of BE and subsequent development of EAC [106].

Nitric oxide (NO) release of the inducible NO-synthetase (iNOS) is another proinflammatory mediator that was found to be related to GERD. Transcript levels of iNOS correlated with the severity of esophagitis, while endothelial NOS (eNOS) and VEGF-A mRNA levels were not affected [107].

NEUROINFLAMMATORY CHANGES IN GERD

As a number of chemical agents may expose to the esophagus during reflux episodes, several chemoreceptors and nerve endings have been started to be characterized. Acid sensitive ion channels (ASIC) have been proposed to carry esophageal sensation and chest pain to the central nervous system. Several receptors have been activated even by stimuli with pH<4 [108]. The Transient Receptor Potential Vanilloid (TRPV)-1 activation is induced by capsaicin and pH drop to pH 5-6. There have been two studies showing the TRPV-1 being expressed on intramucosal C-fibers in human esophagus [109,110]. Besides the pH of the refluxate (acid, weakly acidic and weakly alkaline), the exposure to several other intestinal contents, such as bile acids, intestinal proteases or pancreatic trypsin, have been shown to induce mucosal damage and are suggested to be responsible for the generation of characteristic symptoms [111,112]. Among several putative candidates the proteinase activated receptor-2 (PAR-2) has been proposed for inflammatory and neuroinflammatory epithelial response [113,114]. PAR-2 is specifically activated by serine proteases including trypsin and mast cell-derived tryptase and belongs to the 7-transmembrane G-protein-coupled receptor family. PAR-2 is activated by cleaving the N-terminal sequence of the extracellular receptor domain serving as a tethered ligand [115,116]. PAR-2 activation results in a proinflammatory response in human esophageal cell lines such as IL-8 secretion and COX-2 expression in colonic mucosa [117-119], induces neuroinflammatory effects by releasing substance P (SP) and calcitonin gene related peptide (CGRP) [113], and mediates visceral hypersensitivity and pain [114]. Besides results from colitis models, there has been one study demonstrating elevated PAR-2 expression in human esophageal mucosa of patients with GERD so far, awaiting further results being published [120]. As demonstrated in colitis models, the activation of proteinase activated receptors leads to a sensitization of specific neuronal receptors such as the TRPV-1 and contributes to visceral hypersensitivity [121,122]. Similar results were obtained for mechanical sensations by TRPV-4 activation [123,124] that might explain the genesis of symptoms by mechanical stimuli in patients with GERD. Besides inflammatory and neuroinflammatory effects, the activation of specific receptors by contents of the refluxate, serine proteases such as pancreatic trypsin or tryptase and cathepsin G (released by inflammatory cells) represents a possible pathophysiological mechanism.

CELLS INVOLVED IN GERD-ASSOCIATED INFLAMMATION

Esophageal mucosa harbors epithelial cells, fibroblasts and immune cells, whereas in the submucosa smooth muscle cells and vascular endothelial cells are dominating cells. Rieder *et al.* studied the topical expression of cytokines and their cellular origin. As shown by others IL-1β and IL-6 levels were increased in patients with GERD, but a 5-10 fold differences was noted among samples from upper, middle or lower parts of the esophagus. For both cytokines, highest expression levels were identified in the lower esophagus [82]. Epithelial cells were found to be the major cell type contributing to the release of IL-6 after stimulation with gastric juice. Since the induction of the cytokine was also present after neutralizing the juice to pH 7.4 but was completely abolished after heat-denaturation, proteins and not the acidic pH most likely induce IL-6 expression [82].

Besides paracrine action of cytokines released by immune and epithelial cells, also esophageal circular muscle cells were shown to respond to acidic pH with the release of endogenous platelet activating factor (PAF) that leads to the sequential formation of IL-6, H_2O_2, IL-1β and PAF [125]. The persistent inflammatory condition at esophageal muscle layer is functionally responsible for the reduction of muscle tonus [82,126] leading to impaired LES function as pathophysiological mechanism contributing to GERD [42].

Human esophageal microvascular endothelial cells (HEMEC) were recently analyzed for their contribution to esophageal inflammation. Rafiee *et al.* showed a cytokine release after stimulation by acidic pH that lead to an activation of JNK and subsequent induction of NFκB PI3K/Akt- and MAPKs-pathways [127]. TNF-alpha/LPS activation of HEMEC resulted in upregulation of the cell adhesion molecules (CAM) ICAM-1, VCAM-1, E-selectin, and mucosal addressin CAM-1 (MAdCAM-1), increased IL-8 production, and enhanced leukocyte binding. The induction of VCAM-1 was also caused by acidic exposure of HEMEC supporting the hypothesis that these cells actively respond to abnormal reflux and could contribute to selective recruitment of leukocytes to the esophageal mucosa in the course of GERD [128].

Furthermore, mast cells have been implicated in the pathogenesis of GERD-associated esophagitis. Using a mast cell-deficient mouse model and reconstitution experiments, evidence was provided that mast cells participate in the recruitment of neutrophil granulocytes in reflux-induced esophagitis [129].

ANIMAL MODELS OF GERD – A SHORT OVERVIEW

To perform functional studies and to test new therapies, several animal models were established in rabbits, cats, rats and mice for acute and chronic GERD. GERD is established in these models either by perfusion of acified solutions or surgically by esophagoduodenostomy. Both approaches lead to the development of esophageal erosions and chronic inflammation similar to human disease as shown by several groups [85,129-134]. Most notably, these animal models have been widely used to interfere with molecular pathways identified in human and animal studies. The most investigated ones are the inhibition of oxidative stress by scavengers of ROS to reduce mucosal injury

[125,135,136] and the application of COX-2 inhibitors for the reduction of acute inflammation and prevention of subsequent carcinogenesis [137-139].

GERD-related animal models contribute significantly to the understanding of pathogenesis and provide a suitable tool for novel therapeutic strategies. In addition to manuscripts cited in this paragraph, several articles provide an overview in this field [44,117,140-142].

GENE POLYMORPHISMS OF INFLAMMATORY GENES AND GERD

After the unraveling of the human genome and the identification of multiple genetic variants (mostly single nucleotide polymorphism, SNP) for each gene, it has become clear that the genetic variability contributes significantly to physiology and the development of diseases [143,144]. The pathophysiological relevance of gene polymorphisms depends on the location and their functional effects (e.g. frame shift, premature termination of translation). Well known are SNPs with immediate phenotypic effects leading to hereditary diseases such as Wilson's disease [145]. However, the majority of SNPs has indirect effects leading to changes in protein expression levels or modified interaction of protein or cellular networks. For instance, the mutation of the FOXP3 gene, an essential transcription factor for the development of regulatory T cells, causes the fatale X-linked immune dysregulation, polyendocrinopathy, enteropathy, X-linked syndrome (IPEX) [146]. This fatale monogenetic disorder is accompanied by high incidences of other autoimmune diseases including type 1 diabetes, inflammatory bowel disease and severe allergy [147]. However, most of the genetic variants do not cause immediate pathophysiological effects or a specific disease, but might lead to higher susceptibility for a disease in context to other confounding factors [148]. In the last decade, thousands of these genetic polymorphisms have been linked to the presence of diseases affecting all organs, and novel associations are reported every day. In this context several polymorphisms, in particular cytokine-associated SNPs, were studied in relation to GERD. In focus of most studies was the *IL-1* locus that has been previously linked to gastric carcinogenesis [149]. The identified polymorphism consisted of C-T and T-C transitions at positions −511 and −31 of the *IL-1B* gene, respectively as well as the presence of a penta-allelic tandem repeat in intron 2 of the *IL-1 receptor antagonist* gene (*IL-1RN*) [149]. The combination of both, *IL-1B-511T* haplotype and allele 2 of *IL-1 receptor antagonist* gene (*IL-1RN*2*) resulted in an additive effect leading to an odds ratio of 5.3 (95%CI, 1.9-14) for the likelihood to develop gastric cancer. This genotype is thought to be associated with higher mucosal IL-1β levels leading to gastritis and a subsequent reduction of acid-producing parietal cells with corpus atrophy as indicator lesion of histomorphological transdifferentiation towards intraepithelial neoplasia and gastric adenocarcinoma [150]. Regarding the central pathophysiological role of acid secretion for the development of GERD, it is not surprising that these polymorphisms were studied in context to GERD. It is notable that most epidemiological studies have revealed inverse association between *H. pylori* infection, in particular CagA-positive strains, and the presence of GERD [151,152]. The findings of most studies are in line with this clinical observation. Analyzing 383 patients without gastric cancer and peptic ulcer from Brasil, Queiroz *et al.* showed that among the 98 patients with GERD the *IL-1B-31/C/C* and the *IL1RN*2* were inversely associated to the presence of GERD [153]. Due the almost 100% linkage disequilibrium between *IL-1B-511T/T* and *IL-1B-31C/C*, the identified genotype combination corresponds to the "proinflammatory genotype" introduced by El-Omar that was linked to hypochloridic conditions in the stomach [150]. Since low-acid secretion is naturally a protective effect for the development of GERD, the frequencies of the "*IL-1B* proinflammatory genotype" is reduced in subjects with GERD, because it mediates a protective effect via inducing hypochloridia [153]. Similar results were shown for Japanese patients. Among *H. pylori*-infected subjects, homozygous carriers of the proinflammatory allele *IL-1B-511T/T* had a significantly lower risk for erosive esophagitis (ERD) and GERD-related symptoms compared to those bearing the *IL-1B-511C/C* allele [154].

However, the inverse association between "proinflammatory genotypes" and GERD depends strongly on the presence of *H. pylori* infection. If this infection is not present, the same "proinflammatory genotype" is associated with a higher risk for esophagitis [155]. In Finish patients who underwent endoscopy due to dyspeptic symptoms, the hazard ratio of the *IL-1B-511T/T* + *IL1RN*2* alleles for having ERD were about 4.5 (95% CI: 1.4 – 14.5, P=0.012) compared to those without esophagitis [155]. An important confounding factor in genomic studies is differences in the frequencies of variants among ethnic groups, which has been extensively studied for *IL-1β*

[156,157]. Data, which in part are contradictory to those discussed above, might have their origin in these ethnicity-related issues. In Indian patients, Chourasia *et al.* studied prospectively 144 patients with GERD with respect to endoscopic features, 24h pH metry, *IL-1β* polymorphisms and mucosal expression of IL-1β. Similar to Queiroz *et al.* [153] and Ando *et al.* [154], they identified a protective effect of a "T1 haplotype" (*IL-1B-511T + IL1RN*1*) against GERD among *H. pylori*-positive patients [158]. Interestingly, this haplotype was associated with the highest gastric IL-1B levels, whereas in other ethnic groups, the IL1RN*2 allele is linked to higher IL-1β expression levels [159]. Furthermore, a Japanese study identified the *IL-1B-511T* allele as risk factor for ERD, which was linked to hyperacidity, but the *H. pylori* status was not addressed [160]. Besides *IL-1B* gene polymorphisms, other cytokine genes were studied, but most of them (e.g. *TNF-α-238, IL-4R-1902 and IL-10+1082*) were not associated with the presence of GERD in general [154,161]. However, *IL-10+1082 allele 2* as well as *IL1RN+2018 allele 2* were significantly increased in patients with Barrett's esophagus compared to those with esophagitis [161]. IL-23 receptor (IL-23R) +1142G/A variants were recently identified as another risk factor for the development of Barrett's esophagus. Carriers of the +1142A allele had a 6.8-fold increased risk to have Barrett's esophagus compared to healthy controls, whereas no association between this variant and ERD and NERD was identified [162]. Functionally, the IL-23R modulates STAT-3 pathway that has been linked to the regulation of inflammation-related apoptosis resistance [162]. In contrast to the "Th2-profile" in BE [72], Moons *et al.* identified a genetic profile predisposing to a strong pro-inflammatory host response, mediated by IL-12p70 and partially dependent on IL-10, as risk factor for the development of BE in coincidence with hiatal hernia [163].

NOVEL DIRECTIONS IN GERD-ASSOCIATED INFLAMMATION

Yang *et al.* characterized recently the esophageal microbiome in relation to inflammation and presence of BE and identified two main types [164]. The type I microbiome was dominated by Streptococcus spec. that made up 76% of all identified clones and was identified in 11out of 12 reflux-negative controls. The proportion of this genus was decreased in GERD and BE to

50.5% and 54.1%, respectively. The second microbiome consisted mostly of gram-negative bacteria and anaerobic / microaerophilic species that represented 61.1% of all clones analyzed, while these species made up only 16.1% in the type I microbiome. The Microbiome II was predominantly present in GERD and BE (12 out of 22 patients). It remains unresolved whether the different microbiomes are an independent risk factor for GERD, or it rather is a consequence of an existing disease [164].

It is an established view that the luminal exposure of gastric or gastroduodenal refluxate leads to cellular damage and subsequent inflammation in the esophageal mucosa. The extent of these alterations determines the degree of alterations in the deeper layers of the esophageal tissue. Recently, Souza *et al.* proposed another alternative concept by showing that in a rat model, the release of cytokines by epithelial cells is the initial trigger for the infiltration of immune cells that started in the lamina propria already after 1 week. Spreading of this inflammation into the epithelial layer was observed after 3 weeks [165]. Parallel to the infiltration of the esophageal mucosa at week 3, typical histomorphological alterations such as basal cell hyperplasia and elongation of papilla as well as the appearance of erosions were noted for the first time. Based on this concept, esophagitis represents the initial trigger of GERD-associated histomorphological alterations and is not just secondary to the tissue damage caused by the refluxate [165]. Since similar studies in humans are impossible, it remains unclear at this moment whether this hypothesis relates to GERD in humans.

CONCLUSIONS

The immunological characteristics of esophagitis illustrate a predominant Th1-related pattern for patients with ERD and NERD, while the development of Barrett's metaplasia is linked to a more Th2-directed immune response. Pathophysiologically, the molecular pattern of esophagitis seems to be involved in the development of different GERD-related diseases and complications. Whether some of the identified differences in gene expression patterns can be used as future biomarker for diagnosis, prediction of treatment or surveillance in relation to esophageal carcinogenesis needs further investigations. So far, clinical and functional investigations in combination with endoscopic and histopathological evaluation are the key approaches/techniques for the clinical management of GERD.

REFERENCES

[1] Dent J, El-Serag HB, Wallander MA, Johansson S. Epidemiology of gastro-oesophageal reflux disease: a systematic review. *Gut* 2005: 54, 710-717.

[2] el-Serag HB. Time trends of gastroesophageal reflux disease: a systematic review. *Clin Gastroenterol Hepatol* 2007: 5, 17-26.

[3] Koelz HR, Blum AL, Modlin IM. Costs of Gerd: facts and fiction. *Gastroenterology* 2003: 125, 981-982.

[4] Savarino V, Savarino E, Parodi A, Dulbecco P. Functional heartburn and non-erosive reflux disease. *Dig Dis* 2007: 25, 172-174.

[5] Vakil N, van Zanten SV, Kahrilas P, Dent J, Jones R; Global Consensus Group. The Montreal definition and classification of gastroesophageal reflux disease: a global evidence-based consensus. *Am J Gastroenterol* 2006: 101, 1900-1920.

[6] Wiklund I. Review of the quality of life and burden of illness in gastroesophageal reflux disease. *Dig Dis* 2004: 22, 108-114.

[7] Kulig M, Leodolter A, Vieth M, Schulte E, Jaspersen D, Labenz J, Lind T, Meyer-Sabellek W, Malfertheiner P, Stolte M, Willich SN. Quality of life in relation to symptoms in patients with gastro-oesophageal reflux disease-- an analysis based on the ProGERD initiative. *Aliment Pharmacol Ther* 2003: 18, 767-776.

[8] Rothenberg ME. Biology and treatment of eosinophilic esophagitis. *Gastroenterology* 2009: 137, 1238-49.

[9] Ronkainen J, Aro P, Storskrubb T, Johansson SE, Lind T, Bolling-Sternevald E, Graffner H, Vieth M, Stolte M, Engstrand L, Talley NJ, Agréus L. High prevalence of gastroesophageal reflux symptoms and esophagitis with or without symptoms in the general adult Swedish population: a Kalixanda study report. *Scand J Gastroenterol* 2005: 40, 275-285.

[10] Sharma P, Dent J, Armstrong D, Bergman JJ, Gossner L, Hoshihara Y, Jankowski JA, Junghard O, Lundell L, Tytgat GN, Vieth M. The development and validation of an endoscopic grading system for

Barrett's esophagus: the Prague C & M criteria. *Gastroenterology* 2006: 131, 1392-1399.

[11] Jankowski JA, Provenzale D, Moayyedi P. Esophageal adenocarcinoma arising from Barrett's metaplasia has regional variations in the west. *Gastroenterology* 2002: 122, 588-590.

[12] Yousef F, Cardwell C, Cantwell MM, Galway K, Johnston BT, Murray L. The incidence of esophageal cancer and high-grade dysplasia in Barrett's esophagus: a systematic review and meta-analysis. *Am J Epidemiol* 2008: 168, 237-249.

[13] Long JD, Orlando RC. Nonerosive reflux disease. *Minerva Gastroenterol Dietol*. 2007: 53, 127-141.

[14] Labenz J, Nocon M, Lind T, Leodolter A, Jaspersen D, Meyer-Sabellek W, Stolte M, Vieth M, Willich SN, Malfertheiner P. Prospective follow-up data from the ProGERD study suggest that GERD is not a categorial disease. *Am J Gastroenterol* 2006: 101, 2457-2462.

[15] Nocon M, Labenz J, Jaspersen D, Leodolter A, Richter K, Vieth M, Lind T, Malfertheiner P, Willich SN. Health-related quality of life in patients with gastro-oesophageal reflux disease under routine care: 5-year follow-up results of the ProGERD study. *Aliment Pharmacol Ther*. 2009: 29, 662-668.

[16] Sifrim D, Holloway R. Transient lower esophageal sphincter relaxations: how many or how harmful? *Am J Gastroenterol* 2001: 96, 2529-2532.

[17] Rohof WO, Hirsch DP, Boeckxstaens GE. Pathophysiology and management of gastroesophageal reflux disease. *Minerva Gastroenterol Dietol*. 2009: 55, 289-300.

[18] Jacobson DC, Somers SC, Fuchs CS, Kelly CP, Camargo CA Jr. Body-mass index and symptoms of gastroesophageal reflux in women. *N Engl J Med* 2006: 354, 2340-2348.

[19] Hampel H, Abraham NS, el-Serag HB. Meta-analysis: obesity and the risk for gastroesophageal reflux disease and its complications. *Ann Intern Med* 2005: 143, 199-211.

[20] Ruigómez A, García Rodríguez LA, Wallander MA, Johansson S, Graffner H, Dent J. Natural history of gastro-oesophageal reflux disease diagnosed in general practice. *Aliment Pharmacol Ther* 2004: 20, 751-760.

[21] Ruigomez A, Garcia Rodriguez LA, Wallander MA, et al. Natural history of gastro-oesophageal reflux disease diagnosed in general practice. *Aliment Pharmacol Ther* 2004: 20, 751-760.

[22] Malfertheiner P, Peitz U. The interplay between Helicobacter pylori, gastro-oesophageal reflux disease, and intestinal metaplasia. *Gut.* 2005: 54 (Suppl 1), i13-20.

[23] Malfertheiner P, Megraud F, O'Morain C, Bazzoli F, El-Omar E, Graham D, Hunt R, Rokkas T, Vakil N, Kuipers EJ. Current concepts in the management of Helicobacter pylori infection: the Maastricht III Consensus Report. *Gut* 2007: 56, 772-781.

[24] Bowrey DJ, Williams GT, Carey PD, Clark GW. Inflammation at the cardio-oesophageal junction: relationship to acid and bile exposure. *Eur J Gastroenterol Hepatol.* 2003: 15, 49-54.

[25] Peitz U, Vieth M, Malfertheiner P. Carditis at the interface between GERD and Helicobacter pylori infection. *Dig Dis* 2004: 22, 120-125.

[26] Morini S, Zullo A, Hassan C, Lorenzetti R, Stella F, Martini MT. Gastric cardia inflammation: role of Helicobacter pylori infection and symptoms of gastroesophageal reflux disease. *Am J Gastroenterol.* 2001: 96, 2337-40.

[27] Barlow WJ, Orlando RC. The pathogenesis of heartburn in nonerosive reflux disease: a unifying hypothesis. *Gastroenterology* 2005: 128, 771-778.

[28] Dean BB, Gano AD Jr, Knight K, Ofman JJ, Fass R. Effectiveness of proton pump inhibitors in nonerosive reflux disease. *Clin Gastroenterol Hepatol* 2004: 2, 656-664.

[29] Smith JL, Opekun AR, Larkai E, Graham DY.Sensitivity of the esophageal mucosa to pH in gastroesophageal reflux disease. *Gastroenterology* 1989: 96, 683-689.

[30] Martinez SD, Malagon IB, Garewal HS, Cui H, Fass R. Non-erosive reflux disease (NERD)--acid reflux and symptom patterns. *Aliment Pharmacol Ther.* 2003: 17, 537-545.

[31] Sifrim D, Castell D, Dent J, Kahrilas PJ. Gastro-oesophageal reflux monitoring: review and consensus report on detection and definitions of acid, non-acid, and gas reflux. *Gut* 2004: 53, 1024-1031

[32] Agrawal A, Roberts J, Sharma N, Tutuian R, Vela M, Castell DO. Symptoms with acid and nonacid reflux may be produced by different mechanisms. *Dis Esophagus* 2009: 22, 467-470.

[33] Weigt J, Mönkemüller K, Peitz U, Malfertheiner P. Multichannel intraluminal impedance and pH-metry for investigation of symptomatic gastroesophageal reflux disease. *Dig Dis* 2007: 25, 179-182.

[34] Soderholm JD. Stress-related changes in oesophageal permeability: filling the gaps of GORD? *Gut* 2007: 56, 1177-1180.

[35] Lenglinger J, Eisler M, Riegler M. NERD and "GERD without burn": no more a miracle. *Gastroenterology* 2005: 129, 396-397.

[36] Farré R, De Vos R, Geboes K, Verbecke K, Vanden Berghe P, Depoortere I, Blondeau K, Tack J, Sifrim D. Critical role of stress in increased oesophageal mucosa permeability and dilated intercellular spaces. *Gut* 2007: 56, 1191-1197.

[37] Mönkemüller K, Wex T, Kuester D, Fry LC, Peitz U, Beyer M, Roessner A, Malfertheiner P. Interleukin-1beta and interleukin-8 expression correlate with the histomorphological changes in esophageal mucosa of patients with erosive and non-erosive reflux disease. *Digestion* 2009: 79, 186-195.

[38] Schottenfeld D, Beebe-Dimmer J. Chronic inflammation: a common and important factor in the pathogenesis of neoplasia. *CA Cancer J Clin.* 2006: 56, 69-83.

[39] Abdel-Latif MM, Duggan S, Reynolds JV, Kelleher D. Inflammation and esophageal carcinogenesis. *Curr Opin Pharmacol.* 2009: 9, 396-404.

[40] Carneiro F, Chaves P. Pathologic risk factors of adenocarcinoma of the gastric cardia and gastroesophageal junction. *Surg Oncol Clin N Am.* 2006: 15, 697-714.

[41] Odze RD. Unraveling the mystery of the gastroesophageal junction: a pathologist's perspective. *Am J Gastroenterol.* 2005: 100, 1853-1867.

[42] Orlando RC. Pathophysiology of gastroesophageal reflux disease. *J Clin Gastroenterol* 2008: 42, 584-588.

[43] Malfertheiner P, Hallerbäck B. Clinical manifestations and complications of gastroesophageal reflux disease (GERD). *Int J Clin Pract.* 2005: 59, 346-355.

[44] Barbera M, Fitzgerald RC. Cellular mechanisms of Barrett's esophagus development. *Surg Oncol Clin N Am.* 2009: 18, 393-410.

[45] Michalak J, Bansal A, Sharma P. Screening and surveillance of Barrett's esophagus. *Curr Gastroenterol Rep.* 2009: 11, 195-201.

[46] Zhang HY, Spechler SJ, Souza RF. Esophageal adenocarcinoma arising in Barrett esophagus. *Cancer Lett.* 2009: 275, 170-177.

[47] Ismail-Beigi F, Horton PF, Pope CE 2nd. Histological consequences of gastroesophageal reflux in man. *Gastroenterology* 1970: 58, 163-174.

[48] Hopwood D, Milne G, Logan KR. Electron microscopic changes in human oesophageal epithelium in oesophagitis. *J Pathol.* 1979: 129, 161-167.

[49] Tobey NA, Carson JL, Alkiek RA, Orlando, RC. Dilated intercellular spaces: a morphological feature of acid reflux--damaged human esophageal epithelium. *Gastroenterology*1996: 111, 1200-1205.

[50] Villanacci V, Grigolato PG, Cestari R, Missale G, Cengia G, Klersy C, Rindi G. Dilated intercellular spaces as markers of reflux disease: histology, semiquantitative score and morphometry upon light microscopy. *Digestion.* 2001: 64, 1-8.

[51] Vieth M, Fiocca R, Haringsma J, Delarive J, Wiesel P, Tam W, Tytgat G, Dent J, Edebo A, Lundell L, Stolte M. Radial distribution of dilated intercellular spaces of the esophageal squamous epithelium in patients with reflux disease exhibiting discrete endoscopic lesions. *Dig Dis* 2004: 2, 208-212.

[52] Vieth M, Peitz U, Labenz J, Kulig M, Naucler E, Jaspersen D, Meyer-Sabellek W, Willich S, Lind T, Malfertheiner P, Stolte M. What parameters are relevant for the histological diagnosis of gastroesophageal reflux disease without Barrett's mucosa? *Dig Dis* 2004: 2, 196-201.

[53] Allende DS, Yerian LM. Diagnosing gastroesophageal reflux disease: the pathologist's perspective. *Adv Anat Pathol.* 2009: 16, 161-165.

[54] Marcinkiewicz M, Grabowska SZ, Czyzewska E. Role of epidermal growth factor (EGF) in oesophageal mucosal integrity. *Curr Med Res Opin.* 1998: 14, 145-153.

[55] Calabrese C, Fabbri A, Bortolotti M, Cenacchi G, Areni A, Scialpi C, Miglioli M, Di Febo G. Dilated intercellular spaces as a marker of oesophageal damage: comparative results in gastro-oesophageal reflux disease with or without bile reflux. *Aliment Pharmacol Ther* 2003: 18, 525-532.

[56] Solcia E, Villani L, Luinetti O, Trespi E, Strada E, Tinelli C, Fiocca R. Altered intercellular glycoconjugates and dilated intercellular spaces of

esophageal epithelium in reflux disease. *Virchows Arch* 2000: 436, 207-216.

[57] Malfertheiner P, Mönkemüller K, Wex T. GERD: Endoscopic assessment – a reconciliation with symptoms. *J. Clin. Gastroenterol.* 2007: 41 (Suppl. 2), 193-197.

[58] Asaoka D, Miwa H, Hirai S, Ohkawa A, Kurosawa A, Kawabe M, et al. Altered localization and expression of tight-junction proteins in a rat model with chronic acid reflux esophagitis. *J Gastroenterol.* 2005: 40, 781-790.

[59] Miwa H, Oshima T, Sakurai J, Tomita T, Matsumoto T, Iizuka S, Koseki J. Experimental oesophagitis in the rat is associated with decreased voluntary movement. *Neurogastroenterol Motil.* 2009: 21, 296-303.

[60] Li FY, Li Y. Interleukin-6, desmosome and tight junction protein expression levels in reflux esophagitis-affected mucosa. *World J Gastroenterol.* 2009: 15, 3621-3630.

[61] Jovov B, Van Itallie CM, Shaheen NJ, Carson JL, Gambling TM, Anderson JM, Orlando RC. Claudin-18: a dominant tight junction protein in Barrett's esophagus and likely contributor to its acid resistance. *Am J Physiol Gastrointest Liver Physiol.* 2007: 293, G1106-G1113.

[62] Caviglia R, Ribolsi M, Maggiano N, Gabrielli AM, Emerenziani S, Guarino MPL, Carotti S, Habib FI, Rabitti C, Cicala M. Dilated intercellular spaces of esophageal epithelium in nonerosive reflux disease patients with physiological esophageal acid exposure. *Am J Gastroenterol* 2005: 100, 543-548.

[63] Calabrese C, Bortolotti M, Fabbri A, Areni A, Cenacchi G, Scialpi C, Miglioli M, Di Febo C. Reversibilit of GERD ultrastructural alterations and relief of symptoms after omeprazole treatment. *Am J Gastroenterol* 2005: 100, 537-542.

[64] Haggitt RC. Histopathology of reflux-induced esophageal and supraesophageal injuries. *Am J Med.* 2000: 108 (Suppl 4a), 109S-111S.

[65] Tummala V, Barwick KW, Sontag SJ, Vlahcevic RZ, McCallum RW. The significance of intraepithelial eosinophils in the histologic diagnosis of gastroesophageal reflux. *Am J Clin Pathol.* 1987: 87, 43-48.

[66] Frierson HF Jr. Histological criteria for the diagnosis of reflux esophagitis. *Pathol Annu.* 1992: 27 (Pt 1), 87-104.

[67] Ranatanen TK, Mäkinen JE, Sipponen P, Sihvo E, Leppäniemi A, Salo J. Oesophageal histology in gastroesophageal reflux disease is of minor pre- and postoperative diagnostic value. *Dig Dis* 2004: 2, 202-207.

[68] Zentilin P, Savarino V, Mastracci L, Spaggiari P, Dulbecco P, Ceppa P, Savarino E, Parodi A, Mansi C, Fiocca R. Reassessment of the diagnostic value of histology in patients with GERD, using multiple biopsy sites and an appropriate control group. *Am J Gastroenterol.* 2005: 100, 2299-2306.

[69] Isomoto H, Nishi Y, Kanazawa Y, Shikuwa S, Mizuta Y, Inoue K, Kohno S. Immune and Inflammatory Responses in GERD and Lansoprazole. *J Clin Biochem Nutr.* 2007: 41, 84-91.

[70] Yoshida N, Uchiyama K, Kuroda M, Sakuma K, Kokura S, Ichikawa H, Naito Y, Takemura T, Yoshikawa T, Okanoue T. Interleukin-8 expression in the esophageal mucosa of patients with gastroesophageal reflux disease. *Scand J Gastroenterol.* 2004: 39, 816-822.

[71] Isomoto H, Wang A, Mizuta Y, Akazawa Y, Ohba K, Omagari K, Miyazaki M, Murase K, Hayashi T, Inoue K, Murata I, Kohno S. Elevated levels of chemokines in esophageal mucosa of patients with reflux esophagitis. *Am J Gastroenterol.* 2003: 98, 551-556.

[72] Fitzgerald RC, Onwuegbusi BA, Bajaj-Elliott M, Saeed IT, Burnham WR, Farthing MJ. Diversity in the oesophageal phenotypic response to gastro-oesophageal reflux: immunological determinants. *Gut* 2002: 50, 451-459.

[73] Peitz U, Kouznetsova I, Wex T, Gebert I, Vieth M, Roessner A, Hoffmann W, Malfertheiner P. TFF3 expression at the esophagogastric junction is increased in gastro-esophageal reflux disease (GERD). *Peptides* 2004: 25, 771-775.

[74] Rieder F, Cheng L, Harnett KM, Chak A, Cooper GS, Isenberg G, Ray M, Katz JA, Catanzaro A, O'Shea R, Post AB, Wong R, Sivak MV, McCormick T, Phillips M, West GA, Willis JE, Biancani P, Fiocchi C. Gastroesophageal reflux disease-associated esophagitis induces endogenous cytokine production leading to motor abnormalities. *Gastroenterology* 2007: 132, 154-165.

[75] O'Riordan JM, Abdel-latif MM, Ravi N, McNamara D, Byrne PJ, McDonald GS, Keeling PW, Kelleher D, Reynolds JV. Proinflammatory cytokine and nuclear factor kappa-B expression along the inflammation-

metaplasia-dysplasia-adenocarcinoma sequence in the esophagus. *Am J Gastroenterol.* 2005: 100, 1257-1264.

[76] Kanazawa Y, Isomoto H, Wen CY, Wang AP, Saenko VA, Ohtsuru A, Takeshima F, Omagari K, Mizuta Y, Murata I, Yamashita S, Kohno S. Impact of endoscopically minimal involvement on IL-8 mRNA expression in esophageal mucosa of patients with non-erosive reflux disease. *World J Gastroenterol.* 2003: 9, 2801-2804.

[77] Isomoto H, Kanazawa Y, Nishi Y, Wen CY, Inoue K, Kohno S. Expression of CXC receptor 1 and 2 in esophageal mucosa of patients with reflux esophagitis. *World J Gastroenterol.* 2005: 11, 1793-1797.

[78] Isomoto H, Nishi Y, Kohno S. CXC receptor 1 is overexpressed in endoscopy-negative gastroesophageal reflux disease. *Scand J Gastroenterol.* 2005: 40, 231-232.

[79] Isomoto H, Saenko VA, Kanazawa Y, Nishi Y, Ohtsuru A, Inoue K, Akazawa Y, Takeshima F, Omagari K, Miyazaki M, Mizuta Y, Murata I, Yamashita S, Kohno S. Enhanced expression of interleukin-8 and activation of nuclear factor kappa-B in endoscopy-negative gastroesophageal reflux disease. *Am J Gastroenterol.* 2004: 99, 589-597.

[80] Oh DS, DeMeester SR, Vallbohmer D, Mori R, Kuramochi H, Hagen JA, Lipham J, Danenberg KD, Danenberg PV, Chandrasoma P, DeMeester TR. Reduction of interleukin 8 gene expression in reflux esophagitis and Barrett's esophagus with antireflux surgery. *Arch Surg.* 2007: 142, 554-560.

[81] Isomoto H, Wang A, Nishi Y, Matsumoto A, Shikuwa S, Mizuta Y, Inoue K, Kohno S. Interleukin 8 and 1beta and RANTES levels in esophageal mucosa predict recurrence of endoscopy-negative gastroesophageal reflux disease. *Hepatogastroenterology* 2008: 55, 482-485.

[82] van Roon AH, Mayne GC, Wijnhoven BP, Watson DI, Leong MP, Neijman GE, Michael MZ, McKay AR, Astill D, Hussey DJ. Impact of gastro-esophageal reflux on mucin mRNA expression in the esophageal mucosa. *J Gastrointest Surg.* 2008: 12, 1331-1340.

[83] Corrado G, Zicari A, Cavaliere M, Rea P, Pacchiarotti C, Cerroni F, Pontieri G, Cardi E. Increased release of interleukin-6 by oesophageal mucosa in children with reflux oesophagitis. *Eur J Gastroenterol Hepatol.* 1999: 11, 839-843.

[84]   Nishimoto N, Kishimoto T. Interleukin 6: from bench to bedside. *Nat Clin Pract Rheumatol.* 2006: 2, 619-626.; Erratum in: *Nat Clin Pract Rheumatol.* 2006: 2, 691.

[85]   Li FY, Li Y. Interleukin-6, desmosome and tight junction protein expression levels in reflux esophagitis-affected mucosa. *World J Gastroenterol.* 2009: 15, 3621-3630.

[86]   Naito Y, Kuroda M, Uchiyama K, Mizushima K, Akagiri S, Takagi T, Handa O, Kokura S, Yoshida N, Ichikawa H, Yoshikawa T. Inflammatory response of esophageal epithelium in combined-type esophagitis in rats: a transcriptome analysis. *Int J Mol Med.* 2006: 18, 821-828.

[87]   Dvorak K, Chavarria M, Payne CM, Ramsey L, Crowley-Weber C, Dvorakova B, Dvorak B, Bernstein H, Holubec H, Sampliner RE, Bernstein C, Prasad A, Green SB, Garewal H. Activation of the interleukin-6/STAT3 antiapoptotic pathway in esophageal cells by bile acids and low pH: relevance to barrett's esophagus. *Clin Cancer Res.* 2007: 13(18 Pt 1), 5305-5313.

[88]   Fitzgerald RC, Abdalla S, Onwuegbusi BA, Sirieix P, Saeed IT, Burnham WR, Farthing MJ. Inflammatory gradient in Barrett's oesophagus: implications for disease complications. *Gut* 2002: 51, 316-322.

[89]   Moons LM, Kusters JG, Bultman E, Kuipers EJ, van Dekken H, Tra WM, Kleinjan A, Kwekkeboom J, van Vliet AH, Siersema PD. Barrett's oesophagus is characterized by a predominantly humoral inflammatory response. *J Pathol.* 2005: 207, 269-276.

[90]   Dabbagh K, Takeyama K, Lee HM, Ueki IF, Lausier JA, Nadel JA. IL-4 induces mucin gene expression and goblet cell metaplasia in vitro and in vivo. *J Immunol.* 1999: 162, 6233-6237.

[91]   Taams LS, Palmer DB, Akbar AN, Robinson DS, Brown Z, Hawrylowicz CM. Regulatory T cells in human disease and their potential for therapeutic manipulation. *Immunology* 2003: 118, 1-9.

[92]   Kandulski A, Wex T, Kuester D, Mönkemüller K, Peitz U, Roessner A, Malfertheiner P. Chronic mucosal inflammation of the gastric cardia in gastroesophageal reflux disease is not regulated by FOXP3-expressing T cells. *Dig Dis Sci.* 2009: 54, 1940-1946.

[93]   Kandulski A, Wex T, Kuester D, Peitz U, Gebert I, Roessner A, Malfertheiner P. Naturally occurring regulatory T cells (CD4+,

CD25high, FOXP3+) in the antrum and cardia are associated with higher H. pylori colonization and increased gene expression of TGF-beta1. *Helicobacter* 2008: 13, 295-303.

[94] Tantibhaedhyangkul U, Tatevian N, Gilger MA, Major AM, Davis CM. Increased esophageal regulatory T cells and eosinophil characteristics in children with eosinophilic esophagitis and gastroesophageal reflux disease. *Ann Clin Lab Sci.* 2009: 39, 99-107.

[95] Allameh A, Rasmi Y, Nasseri-Moghaddam S, Tavangar SM, Sharifi R, Sadreddini M. Immunohistochemical analysis of selected molecular markers in esophagus precancerous, adenocarcinoma and squamous cell carcinoma in Iranian subjects. *Cancer Epidemiol.* 2009: 33, 79-84.

[96] Song S, Guha S, Liu K, Buttar NS, Bresalier RS. COX-2 induction by unconjugated bile acids involves reactive oxygen species-mediated signalling pathways in Barrett's oesophagus and oesophageal adenocarcinoma. *Gut* 2007: 56, 1512-1521.

[97] Lurje G, Vallbohmer D, Collet PH, Xi H, Baldus SE, Brabender J, Metzger R, Heitmann M, Neiss S, Drebber U, Holscher AH, Schneider PM. COX-2 mRNA expression is significantly increased in acid-exposed compared to nonexposed squamous epithelium in gastroesophageal reflux disease. *J Gastrointest Surg.* 2007: 11, 1105-1111.

[98] Vallböhmer D, DeMeester SR, Oh DS, Banki F, Kuramochi H, Shimizu D, Hagen JA, Danenberg KD, Danenberg PV, Chandrasoma PT, Peters JH, DeMeester TR. Antireflux surgery normalizes cyclooxygenase-2 expression in squamous epithelium of the distal esophagus. *Am J Gastroenterol.* 2006: 101, 1458-1466.

[99] Abdel-Latif MM, O'Riordan J, Windle HJ, Carton E, Ravi N, Kelleher D, Reynolds JV. NF-kappaB activation in esophageal adenocarcinoma: relationship to Barrett's metaplasia, survival, and response to neoadjuvant chemoradiotherapy. *Ann Surg.* 2004: 239, :491-500.

[100] 100. O'Riordan JM, Abdel-latif MM, Ravi N, McNamara D, Byrne PJ, McDonald GS, Keeling PW, Kelleher D, Reynolds JV. Proinflammatory cytokine and nuclear factor kappa-B expression along the inflammation-metaplasia-dysplasia-adenocarcinoma sequence in the esophagus. *Am J Gastroenterol.* 2005: 100, 1257-1264.

[101] 101. Jenkins GJ, Mikhail J, Alhamdani A, Brown TH, Caplin S, Manson JM, Bowden R, Toffazal N, Griffiths AP, Parry JM, Baxter JN.

Immunohistochemical study of nuclear factor-kappaB activity and interleukin-8 abundance in oesophageal adenocarcinoma; a useful strategy for monitoring these biomarkers. *J Clin Pathol.* 2007: 60, 1232-1237.

[102] 102. Rafiee P, Nelson VM, Manley S, Wellner M, Floer M, Binion DG, Shaker R. Effect of curcumin on acidic pH-induced expression of IL-6 and IL-8 in human esophageal epithelial cells (HET-1A): role of PKC, MAPKs, and NF-kappaB. *Am J Physiol Gastrointest Liver Phy*siol. 2009: 296, G388-G398.

[103] Capello A, Moons LM, Van de Winkel A, Siersema PD, van Dekken H, Kuipers EJ, Kusters JG. Bile acid-stimulated expression of the farnesoid X receptor enhances the immune response in Barrett esophagus. *Am J Gastroenterol.* 2008: 103, 1510-1516.

[104] Grisham MB, Granger DN. Neutrophil-mediated mucosal injury. Role of reactive oxygen metabolites. *Dig Dis Sci.* 1988: 33(3 Suppl), 6S-15S.

[105] Tutar E, Ertem D, Unluguzel G, Tanrikulu S, Haklar G, Celikel C, Ademoglu E, Pehlivanoglu E. Reactive oxygen species and chemokines: are they elevated in the esophageal mucosa of children with gastroesophageal reflux disease? *World J Gastroenterol.* 2008: 14, 3218-3223.

[106] Sihvo EI, Salminen JT, Rantanen TK, Rämö OJ, Ahotupa M, Färkkilä M, Auvinen MI, Salo JA. Oxidative stress has a role in malignant transformation in Barrett's oesophagus. *Int J Cancer.* 2002: 102, 551-555.

[107] Inamori M, Shimamura T, Nagase H, Abe Y, Umezawa T, Nakajima A, Saito T, Ueno N, Tanaka K, Sekihara H, Togawa J, Kaifu H, Tsuboi H, Kayama H, Tominaga S. mRNA expression of inducible nitric oxide synthase, endothelial nitric oxide synthase and vascular endothelial growth factor in esophageal mucosa biopsy specimens from patients with reflux esophagitis. *Hepatogastroenterology* 2006: 53, 361-365.

[108] Holzer P. Taste receptors in the gastrointestinal tract. V. Acid sensing in the gastrointestinal tract. *Am J Physiol Gastrointest Liver Physiol* 2007: 292, G699-G705.

[109] Matthews PJ, Aziz Q, Facer P, Davis JB, Thompson DG, Anand P. Increased capsaicin receptor TRPV1 nerve fibres in the inflamed human oesophagus. *Eur J Gastroenterol Hepatol* 2004: 16, 897-902.

[110] Bhat YM, Bielefeldt K. Capsaicin receptor (TRPV1) and non-erosive reflux disease. *Eur J Gastroenterol Hepatol* 2006: 18, 263-270.

[111] Tack J. Review article: role of pepsin and bile in gastro-oesophageal reflux disease. *Aliment Pharmacol Ther* 2005: 22 (Suppl 1), 48-54.

[112] Sifrim D, Mittal R, Fass R, Smout A, Castell D, Tack J, Gregersen H. Review article: acidity and volume of the refluxate in the genesis of gastro-oesophageal reflux disease symptoms. *Aliment Pharmacol Ther* 2007: 25, 1003-1017.

[113] Steinhoff M, Vergnolle N, Young SH, Tognetto M, Amadesi S, Ennes HS, Trevisani M, Hollenberg MD, Wallace JL, Caughey GH, Mitchell SE, Williams LM, Geppetti P, Mayer EA, Bunnett NW. Agonists of proteinase-activated receptor 2 induce inflammation by a neurogenic mechanism. *Nat Med* 2000: 6, 151-158.

[114] Vergnolle N, Bunnett NW, Sharkey KA, Brussee V, Compton SJ, Grady EF, Cirino G, Gerard N, Basbaum AI, Andrade-Gordon P, Hollenberg MD, Wallace JL. Proteinase-activated receptor-2 and hyperalgesia: A novel pain pathway. *Nat Med* 2001: 7, 821-826.

[115] Scarborough RM, Naughton MA, Teng W, Hung DT, Rose J, Vu TK, Wheaton VI, Turck CW, Coughlin SR. Tethered ligand agonist peptides. Structural requirements for thrombin receptor activation reveal mechanism of proteolytic unmasking of agonist function. *J Biol Chem* 1992: 267, 13146-13149.

[116] Déry O, Corvera CU, Steinhoff M, Bunnett NW. Proteinase-activated receptors: novel mechanisms of signaling by serine proteases. *Am J Physiol* 1998: 274(6 Pt 1), C1429-C1452.

[117] Yoshida N. Inflammation and oxidative stress in gastroesophageal reflux disease. *J Clin Biochem Nutr* 2007: 40, 13-23.

[118] Yoshida N, Katada K, Handa O, Takagi T, Kokura S, Naito Y, Mukaida N, Soma T, Shimada Y, Yoshikawa T, Okanoue T. Interleukin-8 production via protease-activated receptor 2 in human esophageal epithelial cells. *Int J Mol Med* 2007: 19, 335-340.

[119] Cenac N, Coelho AM, Nguyen C, Compton S, Andrade-Gordon P, MacNaughton WK, Wallace JL, Hollenberg MD, Bunnett NW, Garcia-Villar R, Bueno L, Vergnolle N. Induction of intestinal inflammation in mouse by activation of proteinase-activated receptor-2. *Am J Pathol* 2002: 161, 1903-1915.

[120] Inci K, Edebo A, Olbe L, Casselbrant A. Expression of protease-activated-receptor 2 (PAR-2) in human esophageal mucosa. *Scand J Gastroenterol* 2009: 4, 1-8.

[121] Kawao N, Ikeda H, Kitano T, Kuroda R, Sekiguchi F, Kataoka K, Kamanaka Y, Kawabata A. Modulation of capsaicin-evoked visceral pain and referred hyperalgesia by protease-activated receptors 1 and 2. *J Pharmacol Sci* 2004: 94, 277-285.

[122] Dai Y, Moriyama T, Higashi T, Togashi K, Kobayashi K, Yamanaka H, Tominaga M, Noguchi K. Proteinase-activated receptor 2-mediated potentiation of transient receptor potential vanilloid subfamily 1 activity reveals a mechanism for proteinase-induced inflammatory pain. *J Neurosci* 2004: 24, 4293-4299.

[123] Cenac N, Altier C, Chapman K, Liedtke W, Zamponi G, Vergnolle N. Transient receptor potential vanilloid-4 has a major role in visceral hypersensitivity symptoms. *Gastroenterology* 2008: 135, 937-946.

[124] Brierley SM, Page AJ, Hughes PA, Adam B, Liebregts T, Cooper NJ, Holtmann G, Liedtke W, Blackshaw LA. Selective role for TRPV4 ion channels in visceral sensory pathways. *Gastroenterology* 2008: 134, 2059-2069.

[125] Cheng L, Cao W, Behar J, Fiocchi C, Biancani P, Harnett KM. Acid-induced release of platelet-activating factor by human esophageal mucosa induces inflammatory mediators in circular smooth muscle. *J Pharmacol Exp Ther.* 2006: 319, 117-126.

[126] Cheng L, Harnett KM, Cao W, Liu F, Behar J, Fiocchi C, Biancani P. Hydrogen peroxide reduces lower esophageal sphincter tone in human esophagitis. *Gastroenterology* 2005: 129, 1675-1685.

[127] Rafiee P, Ogawa H, Heidemann J, Li MS, Aslam M, Lamirand TH, Fisher PJ, Graewin SJ, Dwinell MB, Johnson CP, Shaker R, Binion DG. Isolation and characterization of human esophageal microvascular endothelial cells: mechanisms of inflammatory activation. *Am J Physiol Gastrointest Liver Physiol.* 2003: 285, G1277-G1292.

[128] Rafiee P, Theriot ME, Nelson VM, Heidemann J, Kanaa Y, Horowitz SA, Rogaczewski A, Johnson CP, Ali I, Shaker R, Binion DG. Human esophageal microvascular endothelial cells respond to acidic pH stress by PI3K/AKT and p38 MAPK-regulated induction of Hsp70 and Hsp27. *Am J Physiol Cell Physiol.* 2006: 291, C931-C945.

[129] Morganstern JA, Wang MY, Wershil BK. Direct evidence of mast cell participation in acute acid-induced esophageal inflammation in mice. *J Pediatr Gastroenterol Nutr.* 2008: 46, 134-138.

[130] Lanas A, Royo Y, Ortego J, Molina M, Sáinz R. Experimental esophagitis induced by acid and pepsin in rabbits mimicking human reflux esophagitis. *Gastroenterology* 1999: 116, 97-107.

[131] Naya MJ, Pereboom D, Ortego J, Alda JO, Lanas A. Superoxide anions produced by inflammatory cells play an important part in the pathogenesis of acid and pepsin induced oesophagitis in rabbits. *Gut* 1997: 40, 175-181.

[132] Babu A, Mauchley D, Meng X, Banerjee AM, Gamboni-Robertson F, Fullerton DA, Weyant MJ. The Secretory Phospholipase A2 Gene is Required for Gastroesophageal Reflux-Related Changes in Murine Esophagus. *J Gastrointest Surg.* 2009: 13, 2212-2218.

[133] Babu A, Meng X, Banerjee AM, Gamboni-Robertson F, Cleveland JC, Damle S, Fullerton DA, Weyant MJ. Secretory phospholipase A2 is required to produce histologic changes associated with gastroduodenal reflux in a murine model. *J Thorac Cardiovasc Surg.* 2008: 135, 1220-1227.

[134] Yamaguchi T, Yoshida N, Tomatsuri N, Takayama R, Katada K, Takagi T, Ichikawa H, Naito Y, Okanoue T, Yoshikawa T. Cytokine-induced neutrophil accumulation in the pathogenesis of acute reflux esophagitis in rats. *Int J Mol Med.* 2005: 16, 71-77.

[135] Hamaguchi M, Fujiwara Y, Takashima T, Hayakawa T, Sasaki E, Shiba M, Watanabe T, Tominaga K, Oshitani N, Matsumoto T, Higuchi K, Arakawa T. Increased expression of cytokines and adhesion molecules in rat chronic esophagitis. *Digestion.* 2003: 68, 189-197.

[136] Inayama M, Hashimoto N, Tokoro T, Shiozaki H. Involvement of oxidative stress in experimentally induced reflux esophagitis and esophageal cancer. *Hepatogastroenterology* 2007: 54, 761-765.

[137] Murphy JO, Ravi N, Byrne PJ, McDonald GS, Reynolds JV. Neither antioxidants nor COX-2 inhibition protect against esophageal inflammation in an experimental model of severe reflux. *J Surg Res.* 2008: 145, 33-40.

[138] Oyama K, Fujimura T, Ninomiya I, Miyashita T, Kinami S, Fushida S, Ohta T, Koichi M. A COX-2 inhibitor prevents the esophageal

inflammation-metaplasia-adenocarcinoma sequence in rats. *Carcinogenesis* 2005: 26, 565-570.

[139] Poplawski C, Sosnowski D, Szaflarska-Popławska A, Sarosiek J, McCallum R, Bartuzi Z. Role of bile acids, prostaglandins and COX inhibitors in chronic esophagitis in a mouse model. *World J Gastroenterol.* 2006: 12, 1739-1742.

[140] Attwood SE, Harrison LA, Preston SL, Jankowski JA. Esophageal adenocarcinoma in "mice and men": back to basics! *Am J Gastroenterol.* 2008: 103, 2367-2372.

[141] Naito Y, Uchiyama K, Kuroda M, Takagi T, Kokura S, Yoshida N, Ichikawa H, Yoshikawa T. Role of pancreatic trypsin in chronic esophagitis induced by gastroduodenal reflux in rats. *J Gastroenterol.* 2006: 41, 198-208.

[142] Hamaguchi M, Fujiwara Y, Takashima T, Hayakawa T, Sasaki E, Shiba M, Watanabe T, Tominaga K, Oshitani N, Matsumoto T, Higuchi K, Arakawa T. Increased expression of cytokines and adhesion molecules in rat chronic esophagitis. *Digestion* 2003: 68, 189-197.

[143] Manolio TA, Collins FS. The HapMap and genome-wide association studies in diagnosis and therapy. *Annu Rev Med.* 2009: 60, 443-456.

[144] Suh Y, Vijg J. SNP discovery in associating genetic variation with human disease phenotypes. *Mutat Res.* 2005: 573, 41-53.

[145] Mak CM, Lam CW. Diagnosis of Wilson's disease: a comprehensive review. *Crit Rev Clin Lab Sci.* 2008: 45, 263-290.

[146] Bennett CL, Christie J, Ramsdell F, Brunkow ME, Ferguson PJ, Whitesell L, Kelly TE, Saulsbury FT, Chance PF and Ochs HD. The immune dysregulation, polyendocrinopathy, enteropathy, X-linked syndrome (IPEX) is caused by mutations of FOXP3. *Nat Genet.* 2001: 27, 20-21.

[147] van der Vliet HJ and Nieuwenhuis EE. PEX as a result of mutations in FOXP3. *Clin Dev Immunol.* 2007: 89017, 2007.

[148] Smith AJ, Humphries SE. Cytokine and cytokine receptor gene polymorphisms and their functionality. *Cytokine Growth Factor Rev.* 2009: 20, 43-59.

[149] El-Omar EM, Carrington M, Chow WH, McColl KE, Bream JH, Young HA, Herrera J, Lissowska J, Yuan CC, Rothman N, Lanyon G, Martin M, Fraumeni JF Jr, Rabkin CS. The role of interleukin-1 polymorphisms in the pathogenesis of gastric cancer. *Nature.* 2001: 412, 99-102.

[150] El-Omar EM, Rabkin CS, Gammon MD, Vaughan TL, Risch HA, Schoenberg JB, Stanford JL, Mayne ST, Goedert J, Blot WJ, Fraumeni JF Jr, Chow WH. Increased risk of noncardia gastric cancer associated with proinflammatory cytokine gene polymorphisms. *Gastroenterology* 2003: 124, 1193-1201.

[151] Souza RC, Lima JH. Helicobacter pylori and gastroesophageal reflux disease: a review of this intriguing relationship. *Dis Esophagus.* 2009: 22, 256-263.

[152] Pereira-Lima JC, Marques DL, Pereira-Lima LF, Hornos AP, Rota C. The role of cagA Helicobacter pylori strains in gastro-oesophageal reflux disease. *Eur J Gastroenterol Hepatol.* 2004: 16, 643-647.

[153] Queiroz DM, Guerra JB, Rocha GA, Rocha AM, Santos A, De Oliveira AG, Cabral MM, Nogueira AM, De Oliveira CA. IL1B and IL1RN polymorphic genes and Helicobacter pylori cagA strains decrease the risk of reflux esophagitis. *Gastroenterology* 2004: 127, 73-79.

[154] Ando T, El-Omar EM, Goto Y, Nobata K, Watanabe O, Maeda O, Ishiguro K, Minami M, Hamajima N, Goto H. Interleukin 1B proinflammatory genotypes protect against gastro-oesophageal reflux disease through induction of corpus atrophy. *Gut* 2006: 55, 158-164.

[155] Koivurova OP, Karhukorpi JM, Joensuu ET, Koistinen PO, Valtonen JM, Karttunen TJ, Niemelä SE, Karttunen RA. IL-1 RN 2/2 genotype and simultaneous carriage of genotypes IL-1 RN 2/2 and IL-1beta-511 T/T associated with oesophagitis in Helicobacter pylori-negative patients. *Scand J Gastroenterol.* 2003: 38, 1217-1222.

[156] Wex T, Bornschein J, Malfertheiner P. Host polymorphisms of immune regulatory genes as risk factors for gastric cancer. *MINERVA Gastroenterologica et Dietologica.* 2009: 55, 395-408.

[157] Schneider BG, Camargo MC, Ryckman KK, Sicinschi LA, Piazuelo MB, Zabaleta J, Correa P, Williams SM. Cytokine polymorphisms and gastric cancer risk: an evolving view. *Cancer Biol Ther.* 2008: 7, 157-162.

[158] Chourasia D, Achyut BR, Tripathi S, Mittal B, Mittal RD, Ghoshal UC. Genotypic and functional roles of IL-1B and IL-1RN on the risk of gastroesophageal reflux disease: the presence of IL-1B-511*T/IL-1RN*1 (T1) haplotype may protect against the disease. *Am J Gastroenterol.* 2009: 104, 2704-2713.

[159] García-González MA, Aísa MA, Strunk M, Benito R, Piazuelo E, Jiménez P, Sopeña F, Lanas A. Relevance of IL-1 and TNF gene polymorphisms on interleukin-1beta and tumor necrosis factor-alpha gastric mucosal production. *Hum Immunol.* 2009: 70, 935-945.

[160] Muramatsu A, Azuma T, Okuda T, Satomi S, Ohtani M, Lee S, Suto H, Ito Y, Yamazaki Y, Kuriyama M. Association between interleukin-1beta-511C/T polymorphism and reflux esophagitis in Japan. *J Gastroenterol.* 2005: 40, 873-877.

[161] Gough MD, Ackroyd R, Majeed AW, Bird NC. Prediction of malignant potential in reflux disease: are cytokine polymorphisms important? *Am J Gastroenterol.* 2005: 100, 1012-1018.

[162] Gaj P, Mikula M, Wyrwicz LS, Regula J, Ostrowski J. Barrett's esophagus associates with a variant of IL23R gene. *Acta Biochim Pol.* 2008: 55, 365-369.

[163] Moons LM, Kusters JG, van Delft JH, Kuipers EJ, Gottschalk R, Geldof H, Bode WA, Stoof J, van Vliet AH, Ketelslegers HB, Kleinjans JC, Siersema PD. A pro-inflammatory genotype predisposes to Barrett's esophagus. *Carcinogenesis* 2008: 29, 926-931.

[164] Yang L, Lu X, Nossa CW, Francois F, Peek RM, Pei Z. Inflammation and intestinal metaplasia of the distal esophagus are associated with alterations in the microbiome. *Gastroenterology* 2009: 137, 588-597.

[165] Souza RF, Huo X, Mittal V, Schuler CM, Carmack SW, Zhang HY, Zhang X, Yu C, Hormi-Carver K, Genta RM, Spechler SJ. Gastroesophageal reflux might cause esophagitis through a cytokine-mediated mechanism rather than caustic acid injury. *Gastroenterology* 2009: 137, 1776-1784.

In: Reflux Disease: Causes, Symptoms and ...   ISBN: 978-1-61668-694-9
Editor: G. M. Esposito, pp. 37-72   © 2010 Nova Science Publishers, Inc.

Chapter II

Systemic Implications in the Pharmacologic Treatment of Gastroesophageal Reflux Disease (GERD)

William A. Paradise[1], Benjamin J. Vesper[1,2],
Kenneth W. Altman[3] and James A. Radosevich[1,2]
[1]University of Illinois at Chicago, Chicago, IL, 60612, USA;
[2]Jesse Brown VAMC, Chicago, IL, 60612, USA;
[3]Mount Sinai School of Medicine, New York, NY, 10029, USA.

ABSTRACT

Gastroesophageal reflux disease (GERD) affects women, men and children across worldwide demographic groups. The occurrence rate has increased over the past few decades, and epidemiological evidence suggests it will continue to do so into the foreseeable future. Left untreated, more serious diseases can result, including esophagitis and/or esophageal cancer. A number of treatment options are currently available for GERD, however the proton pump inhibitors (PPIs) are by far the most common treatment used. PPIs stop production of acid by shutting down the H^+/K^+-ATPase enzyme located in parietal cells. Evidence from recent studies suggests because PPI treatment is systemic, H^+/K^+-ATPase in tissues outside the stomach may also be impacted. These include the upper aerodigestive, otolaryngological, and esophageal regions. The use of PPIs may also be impacting H^+/K^+-ATPase within normally occurring human microbiota populations by raising pH levels, thereby potentially disturbing commensal bacteria and fungi. These colonies normally prevent opportunistic infections. Finally, there are two fundamentally different philosophical approaches chosen for PPI therapy by clinicians. The first pursues short-term treatment only when symptoms are present. The second treats continuously over time, which can lead to a number of undesired side effects. A further concern to clinicians is that while PPIs have been found to heal esophagitis, relapse occurs in the majority of patients shortly after discontinuing treatment. However, there are many negative implications for long-term use of PPIs, which also need to be considered. The impact on patient microbiota may be in ways not yet fully understood and therefore can complicate PPI therapy decisions and choices.

1. INTRODUCION

Gastroesophageal reflux disease (GERD) is a clinically diagnosed condition in which stomach acid is believed to reflux into the esophagus. GERD affects men, women and children. It is a chronic disorder. The most common symptoms of the disease include heartburn and the regurgitation and/or irritation associated with large meal volumes [1]. Symptoms also include chest pain, dysphagia, and coughing [1,2]. Episodes of heartburn and/or acid regurgitation have been found in nearly 20% of Americans and roughly 15% of the worldwide population, occurring as frequently as once a week [3,4]. GERD has increased in the last several decades with recent epidemiological studies suggesting these numbers will continue to rise in the future [5-7].

GERD is often self-diagnosed and treated through use of over-the-counter (OTC) drug therapies. Furthermore, both tablet and intravenous delivery methods are used in the United States and Europe [8,9]. Therefore, many patients suffering from minor cases of GERD rely on therapies based on self-diagnosis. However, in more severe cases, clinical evaluation and treatment is necessary. Commonly used detection techniques for GERD include contrast dyes, upper gastrointestinal endoscopy, catheters and capsules measuring intraesophageal pH, and radiographic examinations [2].

Patients presenting with symptoms of GERD most commonly fall into one of two categories: (a) nonerosive reflux disease (NERD) or (b) erosive esophagitis. NERD is characterized by symptoms of GERD but without mucosal injury as evidenced through upper endoscopy. Swelling and inflammation of the esophagus are typical indicators of erosive esophagitis, which can also include the condition known as Barrett's esophagus. Barrett's esophagus is many times a precursor of esophageal cancer [10]. High body mass index levels and poor lifestyle choices appear to correlate to the disease evolution from Barrett's esophagus to esophageal cancer. Examples of high risk lifestyle factors include alcohol and tobacco consumption and maintaining diets low in fruit [11,12].

There are a variety of options available to patients for the treatment of GERD. The therapy program is usually based upon severity and degree of symptoms. Therapies may range from simple dietary or lifestyle changes in very minor cases, to self-medication with OTC products, to surgery in severe cases. Proton pump inhibitors (PPIs) are among the most readily chosen drug therapy options. This class of drugs targets and regulates gastric acid secretion and transport, thereby relieving symptoms and healing esophageal damage. The PPIs and other drugs used to treat GERD are described in more detail in Section 3.

Once diagnosed, patients typically face two general treatment options [13]; the first is to treat only when symptoms are present. While current therapies are rather effective for the short-term elimination of symptoms, a permanent cure to the disease has yet to be found. As a result, recurrence of the disease is common. The second option is to treat continuously; but this puts the patient at risk for long-term side effects. Because of the issues associated with both short-term and long-term treatment options, new therapies are currently being explored.

Further contributing to the uncertainty surrounding long-term PPI use and the treatment of GERD is the recent discovery of non-gastric human cells containing the H^+/K^+-ATPase enzyme and the known presence of commensal acid-producing bacteria and fungi in the human body [13-19]. It is surprising how little is known about the effects of long-term PPI use on the indigenous human microbiota, given how many of these bacteria and fungi are associated with pH regulation and/or acid production. Recent research has begun to address this area in an effort to better understand GERD.

2. GASTRIC ACID SECRETION

Gastric acid is utilized in the stomach to breakdown proteins and absorb vitamins and minerals. It also plays an important role in preventing opportunistic infection and overgrowth of bacteria and fungi [20].

Acid Production and Regulation

Gastric acid is produced and regulated by an interrelated, physiological pathway. This process includes a series of hormonal, neuronal, and paracrine pathways coordinating stomach activities through both central and peripheral neural systems [21,22]. Parietal cells found on the stomach lining produce gastric acid with up to 50% of all acid production resulting from the vagus nerve directly stimulating parietal cells [23]. Further acid is produced through peripheral mechanisms. These include endocrine cells, both G cells, D cells, and enterochromaffin like (ECL) cells (Figure 1).

Parietal cells play a key role in the production of gastric acid. The basolateral membrane of these cells contains a variety of different receptors which, when activated by the appropriate physiological stimulant, initiate gastric acid production. These various chemical stimuli include gastrin, acetylcholine and histamine. Gastrin is produced by G cells within the antrum; following production, the gastrin is then carried by the blood to ECL cells. Here it binds to cholecystokinin$_2$ (CCK$_2$) receptors, thereby triggering the release of histamine [21,22,24,25]. Histamine release can also be triggered by acetylcholine (Ach), which when released from postganglionic enteric neurons, can attach to the M$_3$ receptors on ECL cells. The histamine then binds to H$_2$ receptor sites in the parietal cells. Alternatively, Ach can bind to M$_3$ receptors on parietal cells, directly stimulating acid secretion [20,22]. The release and subsequent binding of gastrin, acetylcholine and/or histamine act as chemical stimulants generating signals along transduction pathways, which in turn cause an increase in the concentration of intracellular calcium and/or cyclic adenosine monophosphate (cAMP). This increased presence of Ca^{2+} and cAMP results in a distinct morphological transformation which leads to the final step in acid secretion: the release of the enzyme H$^+$/K$^+$-ATPase from cytosolic tubulovesicles into the apical membrane of the parietal cells [21,22,26].

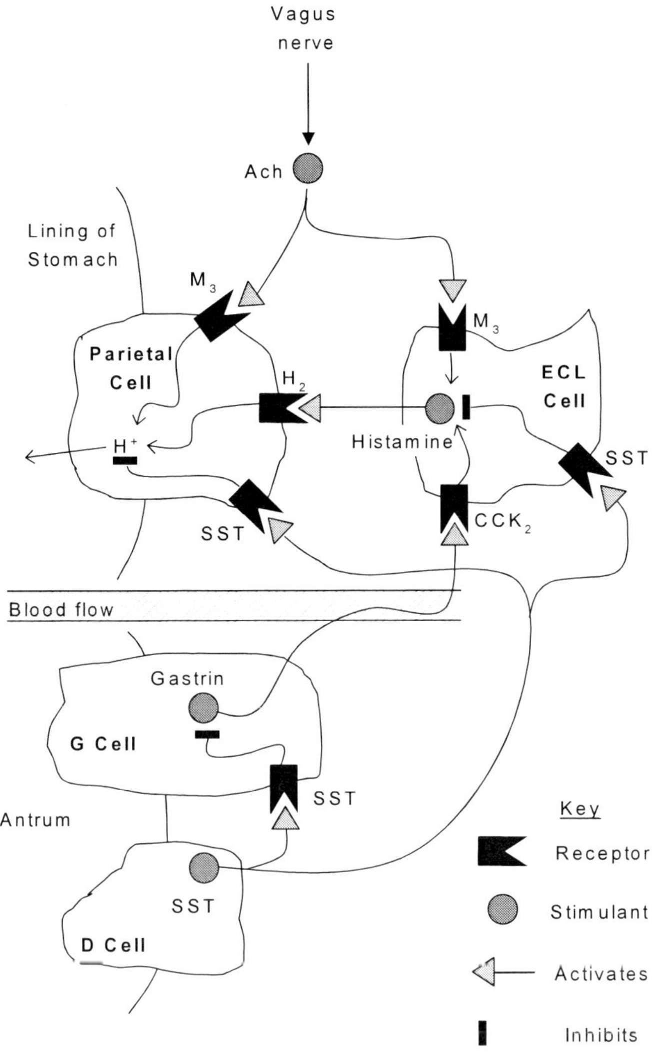

Figure 1. Simplified version of the gastric acid production/secretion pathway. Reproduced with permission [13]. Copyright 2008 Wiley-VCH Verlag GmbH & Co. KGaA, Weinheim.

Once stimulated, the parietal cells release hydrochloric acid (HCl) into the lumen of the stomach via the H^+/K^+-ATPase (Figure 2). This is accomplished by H^+ being transported across the apical membrane and into the canaliculi of the parietal cells in exchange for K^+. Simultaneously, Cl^- is also transported via Cl⁻ channels in the apical membrane, thereby maintaining chemical equilibrium. K^+ is then recycled from the cytoplasm into the canaliculi through potassium channels within the apical membrane. Na^+/K^+-ATPase enzymes located on the basolateral membrane also help regulate the cytoplasmic K^+ concentration. Additionally, for each H^+ transported into the canaliculi via H^+/K^+-ATPase, a HCO_3^{3-} ion is concurrently released from the parietal cell cytoplasm through a basolateral Cl^-/HCO_3^{3-} exchanger, while a Cl⁻ ion is also released into the cytoplasm [21,22,24,26].

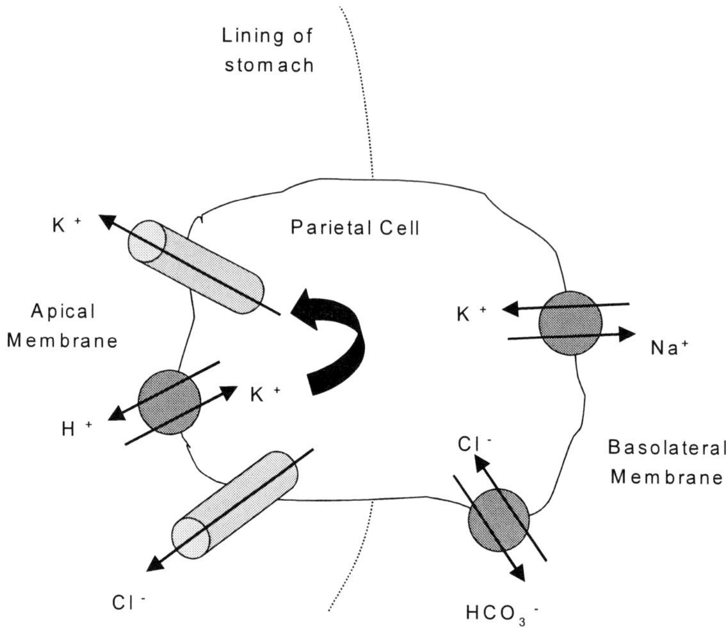

Figure 2. Parietal ion exchange during gastric acid secretion. Reproduced with permission [13]. Copyright 2008 Wiley-VCH Verlag GmbH & Co. KGaA, Weinheim.

The release of H^+ for the production of gastric acid is regulated through an intragastric feedback/control loop. The increased H^+ concentration in the canaliculi of the parietal cells results in a pH of 1.0 or lower, compared with a pH of approximately 7.4 in the cytoplasm of the parietal cell [26,27]. Once the pH of the intragastric acid decreases sufficiently, somatostatin (SST), a peptide, is released from antral D cells in order to stop acid secretion (Figure 1). SST inhibits acid secretion by either directly impacting parietal cells or indirectly inhibiting the release of histamine and gastrin in ECL and G cells, respectively [23]. Endogenous prostaglandins and secretin, a peptide, are also believed to play key roles in acid suppression and regulation, working in tandem to shut down H^+/K^+-ATPase release [24].

Gastric H^+/K^+-ATPase Structure and Properties

H^+/K^+-ATPase is a heterodimer made up of two subunits: α and β (Figure 3). The functionality and structure of each subunit differs as follows. The α subunit is responsible for catalytic processes, transport, and the binding sites for ATP, H^+, and K^+ activity [23,26]. The structure is ten helical transmembrane segments, located mostly within the cytoplasm. The β subunit helps stabilize subunit α and directs the heterodimer to membrane destinations within the cell. The β subunit contains seven N-linked oligosaccharides, is a single transmembrane segment in molecular size, and is predominately extracellular. However it plays a significant role in protecting the H^+/K^+-ATPase from the highly acidic environment of the apical lumen [23].

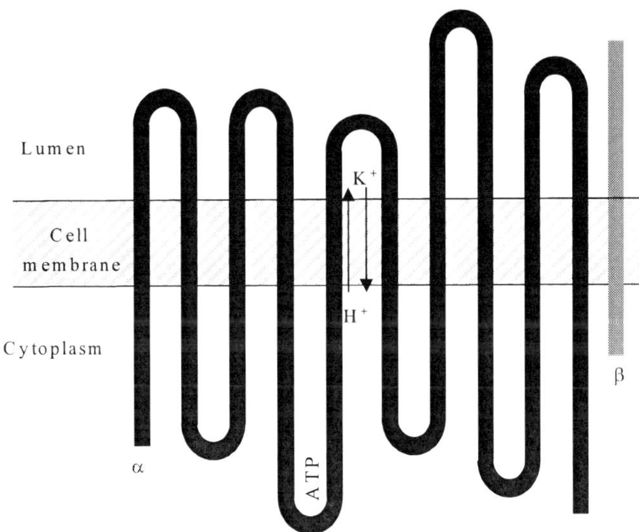

Figure 3. H^+/K^+-ATPase structure. Reproduced with permission [13]. Copyright 2008 Wiley-VCH Verlag GmbH & Co. KGaA, Weinheim.

3. GERD TREATMENT

Given the overall complexity of gastric acid secretion and the many physiological mechanisms involved in the process, as discussed in the previous section, a number of potential therapeutic targets for GERD have already been identified. As such, several classes of GERD drugs exist, either as over-the-counter or prescription medication; each class of drug targets a specific aspect of the gastric acid production/secretion process. Currently available drugs include antacids and alginates, histamine H_2-receptor antagonists (H_2RAs), proton pump inhibitors (PPIs), prokinetics, and potassium-competitive acid blockers (P-CABs). Pre-clinical studies have also looked at a new area of GERD treatment: anti-gastrin agents. We discuss each of these treatment options in more detail here and summarize the various classes of GERD drugs in Table 1 at the end of this section.

Antacids and Alginates

The most commonly taken OTC drugs are antacids and alginates, since prior consultation with a physician is not necessary. These drugs offer local and fast relief from heartburn, but are only short-term solutions to the problem. Antacids work by locally lowering the pH of the stomach and esophagus, while alginates prevent acid from reaching the esophagus by providing a barrier to the top of the stomach. Alginates are typically formulated with antacids to improve efficacy [28]. The most commonly used antacids and alginates are aluminum hydroxide, hydrotalcite, and magaldrate. Side effects resulting from antacid and alginate use is rare given that only very small amounts of the drugs enter circulation; however, because these drugs provide only short-term relief, frequent dosing is necessary. As such, the antacids and alginates are not practical for treating erosive esophagitis, but may be useful in treating minor cases of GERD [28].

Histamine H_2-receptor Antagonists

The histamine H_2-receptor antagonists (H_2RAs)—the first effective treatment for acid-related diseases—are a class of drugs that reversibly block

H_2-receptors on parietal cells, thereby inhibiting acid secretion [29,30]. Figure 4 shows the structures of four H_2RAs: ranitidine, famotidine, cimetidine, and nizatidine. The H_2RAs have a slower onset of action than the antacids, and like the antacids and alginates, H_2RAs provide only short-term relief [31]. Furthermore, pharmacological tolerance to the drug typically develops within 1-2 weeks of use [32], and H_2RAs have not been shown to improve esophagitis healing [33]. Thus, while both OTC and prescription formulations are available for H_2RAs, the drugs are best suited for treating only minor cases of heartburn. Due to these drawbacks, the treatment of GERD has shifted away from the H_2RAs and is currently focused more strongly on the proton pump inhibitors, discussed next.

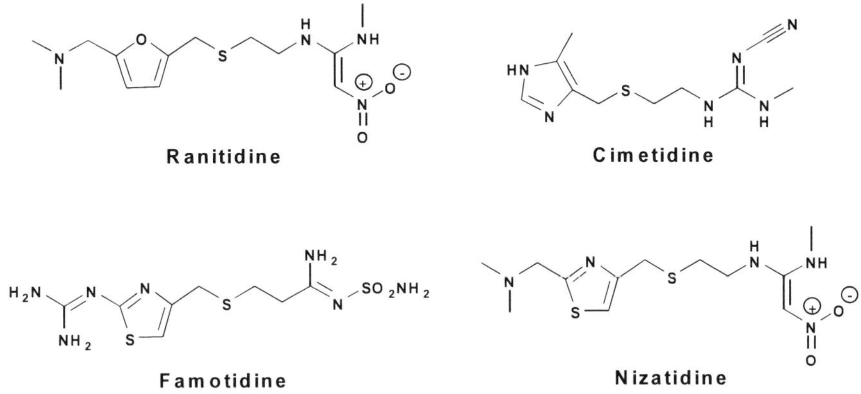

Ranitidine

Cimetidine

Famotidine

Nizatidine

Figure 4. Chemical structures of histamine H_2-receptor antagonists currently in use.

Proton Pump Inhibitors (PPIs)

The PPIs are the most commonly used treatment method for combating moderate-to-severe cases of GERD. Designed as weak bases which react with secreted gastric acid in the stomach to create an active form of the drug (sulphenamide), the PPIs block acid transport by binding to the cysteine residues of the H^+/K^+-ATPase enzyme via irreversible disulfide bonds [22,34,35]. Due to the irreversible nature of the sulphenamide binding, once-daily repeated dosing with currently available PPIs results in increased inhibition of the proton pumps, typically controlling acid secretion within 3-5 days [35]. Figure 5 shows the first-generation PPIs currently available:

lansoprazole, rabeprazole, omeprazole, esomeprazole, and pantoprazole [33,36]. All five PPIs are available in tablet form; within the last decade, three of these—lansoprazole (Prevacid®), pantoprazole (Protonix®), and esomeprazole (Nexium®)—have also been approved for intravenous use in the United States [8,37].

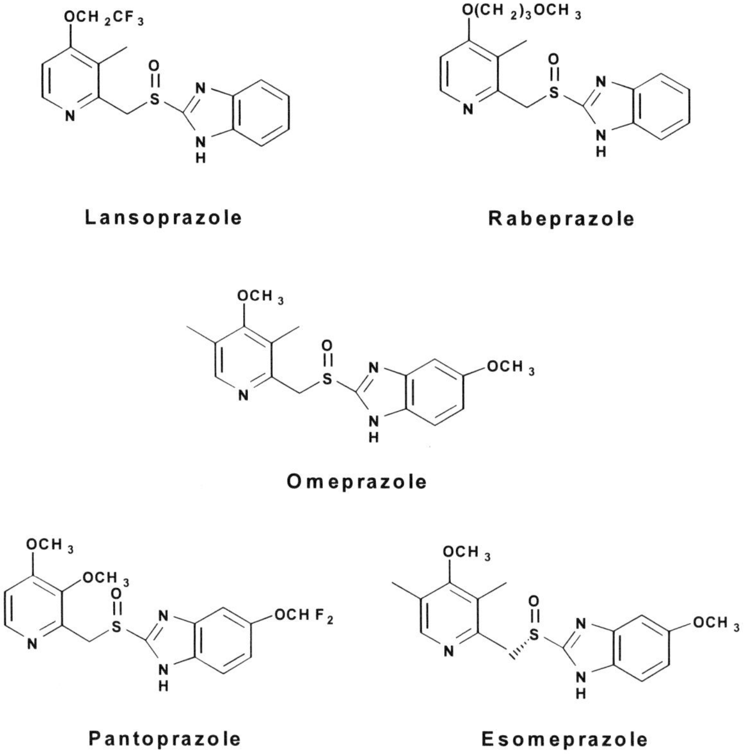

Lansoprazole

Rabeprazole

Omeprazole

Pantoprazole

Esomeprazole

Figure 5. Chemical structures of proton pump inhibitors currently in use.

The PPIs are typically effective in the short-term relief of GERD symptoms, and improved esophageal healing has been reported with long-term PPI use [28]. Further, PPIs are a popular choice with patients since they are typically taken only once per day (although twice per day dosing is sometimes required), and the onset of relief is usually faster than that observed with either the H_2RAs or prokinetics (described next) [28].

Despite these advantages, problems still exist with PPI treatment. Side effects including diarrhea, nausea, headaches, anaphylaxis, and insomnia are sometimes observed with short-term treatment [36,38,39]. Also, the first-generation PPIs in use today are known to exhibit considerable interpatient variability, and adverse interactions with other drugs has been documented in many cases [24]. However, the most complicating problem of PPI use is that the drugs do not completely cure the disease. Rebound acid hypersecretion is often observed after treatment has ended [40], and approximately 80% of patients relapse within 30 weeks after discontinuing use [41]. Additional problems have also been linked to long-term PPI use, including increased disposition to gastrinomas [40], severe hypomagnesaemia [42], and an increase in hip-fracture rates [43]. We document these and other long-term problems in more detail in Section 5.

In an effort to address some of the short-comings associated with PPI use, recent research has focused on two main areas: 1) incorporating the first-generation PPIs into formulations that will enhance the efficacy of the drugs and/or patient compliance, and 2) developing novel PPIs. First, initial work has been carried out on dexlansoprazole MR (also known as TAK-390MR; MR: "modified release"), an enantiomer of lansoprazole that has been formulated as a dual delayed- and extended-release drug. TAK-390MR exhibits higher plasma concentrations and longer acid suppression than conventional PPIs [35,44,45]. Like the traditional PPIs, TAK-390MR was still found to be effective in healing erosive esophagitis and controlling heartburn [46]. Further trials are needed to verify its potential as a future commercial alternative.

While TKA-390MR appears to be the most promising formulation currently under development, a number of other formulations are also being investigated or have recently been introduced into clinical practice. Many of these formulations, such as the lansoprazole orally disintegrating tablet (ODT) and the immediate-release (IR) omeprazole formulation, are designed to increase patient compliance of the current PPIs [24].

Second, two new PPIs are currently being studied in humans (Figure 6). Ilaprazole (IY-81149) is a benzimidazole derivative currently marketed in Asia, but it has not yet completed clinical trials in the United States [24]. *In vivo* rat studies found that ilaprazole blocked acid secretion more effectively and for a longer period of time than omeprazole [47]. Initial studies of ilaprazole in GERD patients confirmed these results [48]. Tenatoprazole (TU-199), in contrast to ilaprazole and the other PPIs currently available, is not a benzimidazole derivative, but rather is made up of a pyridine ring linked to an imidazopyridine ring via a sulfinyl-methyl bond. In the first human trials of tenatoprazole, a study in Japan (n=6) showed that the drug had a half-life 7-fold longer than that of other PPIs, resulting in a long-lasting antisecretory effect from a single dose [24,49]. A later study involving a small number of Causasians (n=8) revealed similar results [50,51]. While the early results are promising, randomized, controlled clinical trials involving a larger sample size still need to be performed [35].

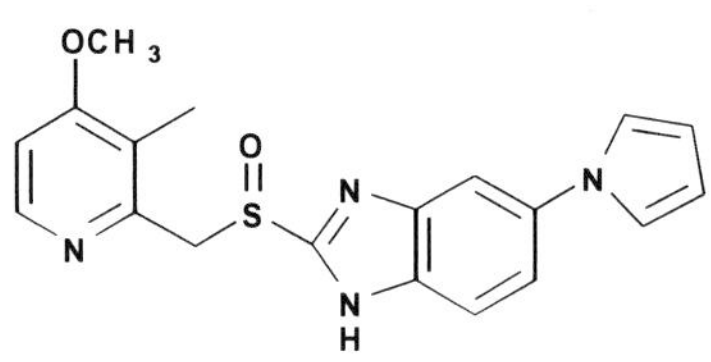

Ilaprazole (IY-81149) 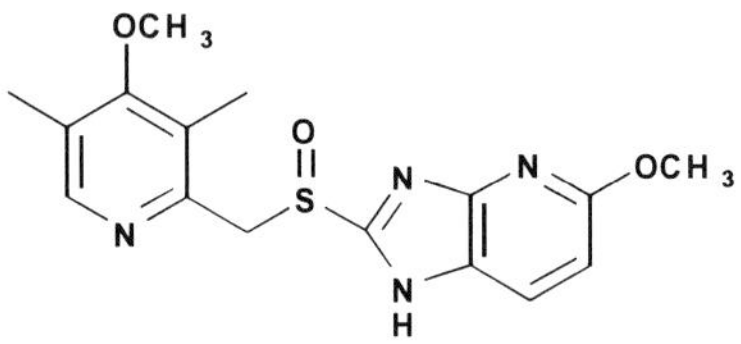   **Tenatoprazole (TU-199)**

Figure 6. Chemical structures of proton pump inhibitors currently under development.

Prokinetics

The prokinetics are a class of drug designed to release the stomach contents and increase esophageal clearance. They activate serotonin 5-hydroxytryptamine 4 (5-HT$_4$) receptors and/or act directly on dopaminergic receptors in the stomach to agonistically release acetylcholine. These drugs behave similarly to the H$_2$RAs: they provide effective short-term acid suppression, but the onset of relief is much slower than that found with antacids. Furthermore, relief typically lasts for only 4-8 hours, meaning that patients often take two doses per day [28]. Additionally, numerous side effects have been associated with prokinetics use, including fatigue, parkinsonism, tardive dyskinesia, tremor, and cardiac events. The drugs have also not been found to improve high-grade esophagitis [28,33]. Thus, prokinetics are typically only useful for minor cases of GERD and therefore are not often prescribed.

Figure 7 shows three first-generation prokinetic drugs (metoclopramide, domperidone, and cisapride) and ATI-7505, a new prokinetic currently in development. Metoclopramide has been used clinically for over three decades in the treatment of GERD symptoms, particularly in pediatric care [52], despite having been shown to cause adverse neurological symptoms due to the drug crossing the blood-brain barrier [52-54]. In contrast to metoclopramide, domperidone exhibits little penetration of the blood-brain barrier and, due to its efficacy and safer profile, was recently approved for use in the United States [54,55]. The prokinetic cisapride, despite its ability to reduce acid reflux entering the esophagus, has been linked to fatal arrhythmias and was subsequently discontinued in both Europe and the United States [35]. Initial studies of ATI-7505 have shown the drug to exhibit similar pharmacology to that of cisapride [56]; but unlike cisapride, Phase II clinical studies have shown that ATI-7505 is safe in humans. The drug is expected to advance to late-stage clinical trials [57].

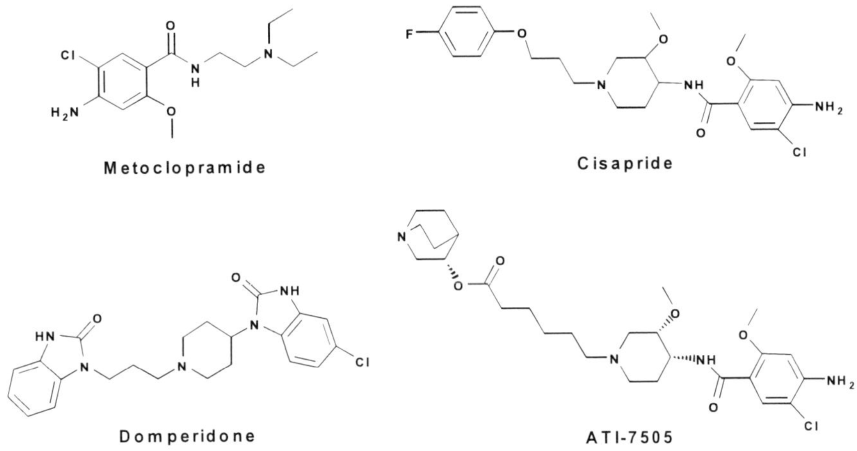

Figure 7. Chemical structures of the prokinetics currently in use or under development.

Potassium-Competitive Acid Blockers (P-CABs)

The P-CABs, also known as acid pump antagonists, are a class of drugs that inhibit acid secretion by reversibly binding to the K^+-binding domain of parietal H^+/K^+-ATPase. There are currently four classes of P-CABs—imidazopyridines, pyrimidines, quinolines, and imidazonaphthyridine—as shown in Figure 8. Despite differences in structure, the mechanism by which each class blocks acid is the same [26,58]. In general, the P-CABs offer fast relief at a single dose (typically within 30 minutes of administration) and without the development of tolerance [35]. Members of the P-CABs include revaprazan (YH1885), soraprazan (BY359), AZD0865, and PF-03716556 (Figure 9). While revaprazan is currently commercially available [59], both soraprazan and AZD0865 have recently been dropped from development following Phase II clinical studies [26,35]. Pre-clinical results for PF-03716556 have been promising, however, as the drug was found to have a greater potency than revaprazan and a faster onset then the commercially available PPI omeprazole [59].

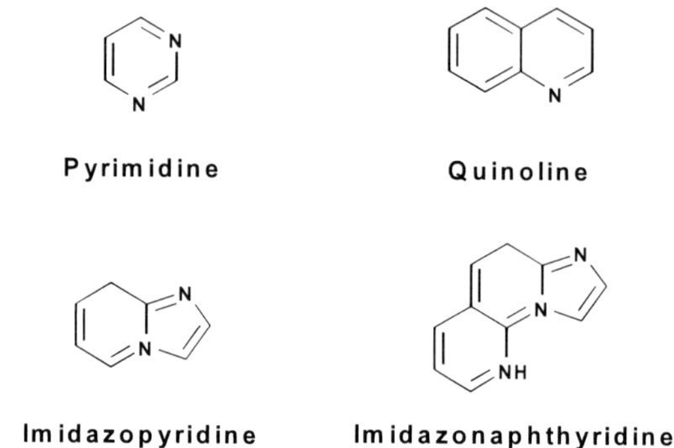

Figure 8. The four classes of potassium competitive acid blockers.

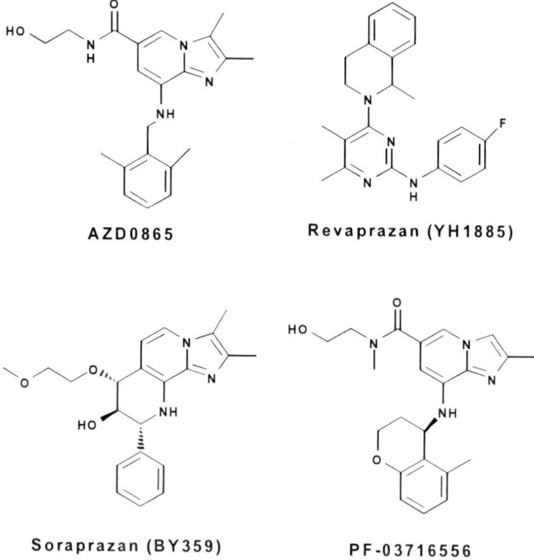

Figure 9. Chemical structures of potassium competitive acid blockers previously studied or currently in use/under development.

Anti-gastrin Agents

A relatively new area of GERD treatment involves trying to block gastrin-mediated acid secretion. While the cholecystokinin$_2$ (CCK$_2$) receptor antagonists drugs have garnered the most research in this area to date, work has also been performed on an anti-gastrin vaccine.

CCK$_2$ Receptor Antagonists

The CCK$_2$ receptor antagonists are a class of drugs targeting the CCK$_2$ receptors on ECL cells and acid-secreting parietal cells [60]. While gastrin can affect both ECL cells and parietal cells, it is believed to have a far greater effect on the former [24]. Therefore, successfully blocking the CCK$_2$ receptors on ECL cells would likely result in a reduction of histamine production, thereby reducing overall acid production. Indeed, initial clinical trials of the first-generation CCK$_2$ receptor antagonist spiroglumide (CR-02194) showed a reduction in gastrin-induced acid secretion [61]. However, it has been discontinued due to a lack of potency. Likewise, another first-generation CCK$_2$ agent, YF-476, was found to reduce acid secretion in humans, but this drug has also since been discontinued, due to a development of tolerance in patients [24].

Spiroglumide and YF-476 are members of the two subclasses of CCK$_2$ receptor antagonist agents prepared to date: amino acid derivatives (Figure 10) and benzodiazepine derivatives (Figure 11), respectively. Second-generation candidates from each of the two subclasses have subsequently been prepared, and initial studies have yielded favorable results. Itriglumide (CR-2945), an amino acid derivative, exhibited good oral bioavailability and greater potency than both omeprazole and ranitidine in pre-clinical studies [62], and showed a dose-dependent inhibition of gastrin-stimulated acid secretion in a follow-up study in humans [63]. Likewise, the CCK$_2$ agent Z-360, a benzodiazepine, was found to block acid secretion in pre-clinical studies: 70% of postprandial acid secretion was inhibited in Pavlov pouch dogs [64].

Despite the promising early results obtained to date for the second-generation agents, it is widely believed that the CCK$_2$ receptor antagonists will have to be used in combination with the PPIs in order to be a viable treatment option for GERD patients [24,26]. In addition to the tolerance observed with spiroglumide mentioned above, it is thought that CCK$_2$ antagonists may delay mucosal healing [24]. However, when used in combination with PPIs, early research has suggested that the CCK_2 receptor antagonists may reduce omeprazole-induced hyperplasia [64]. Furthermore, CCK_2 receptors have been identified in a number of tumors types throughout the body, including GI tumors, suggesting the CCK_2 antagonists may be useful as anti-cancer drugs [65]. To this end, recent research found that Z-360 exhibits anti-tumor properties in a hepatic metastasis model [66].

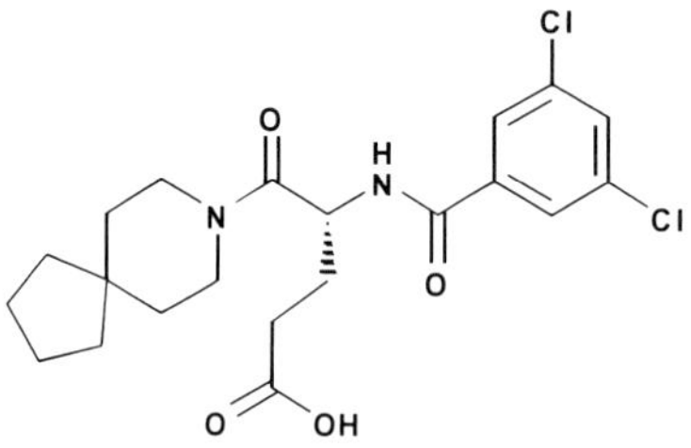

Spiroglumide (CR-02194)

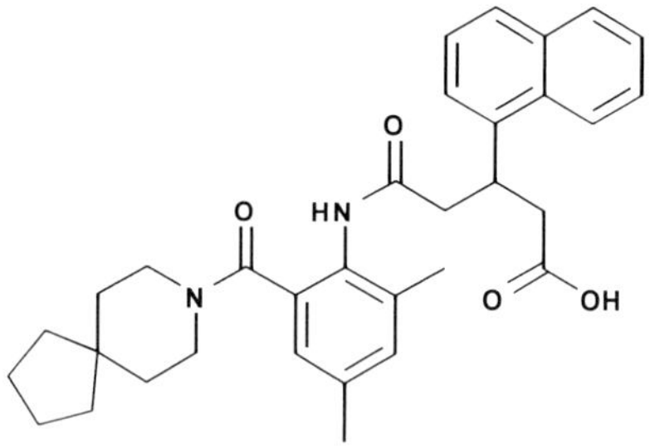

Itriglumide (CR-2945)

Figure 10. Chemical structures of cholecystokinin$_2$ receptor antagonists belonging to the amino acid derivative subclass.

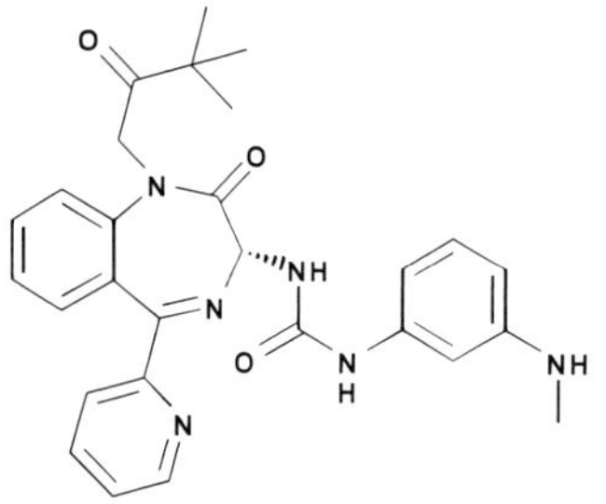

YF-476

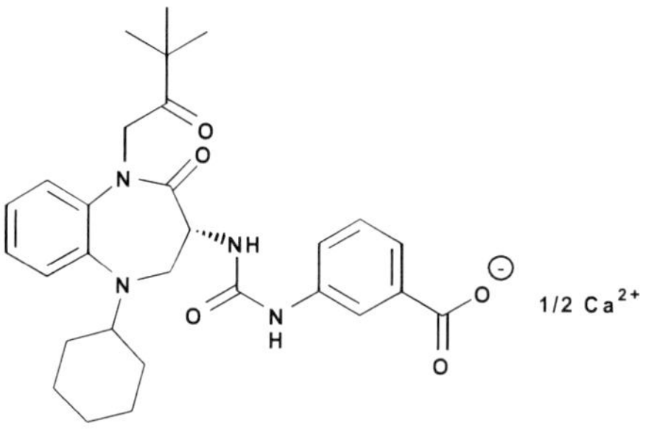

Z-360

Figure 11. Chemical structures of cholecystokinin$_2$ receptor antagonists belonging to the benzodiazepine derivative subclass.

Table 1. Comparative Overview of Current GERD Treatment Options

Drug Class/Types	Key Therapy Attributes
1. Proton Pump Inhibitors (PPIs) Omeprazole Lansoprazole Rabeprazole Pantoprazole Esomeprazole Ilaprazole Tenatoprazole	- React with cysteine residues to permanently block H^+/K^+-ATPase - Improves healing of esophagus - Systemic - OTC and prescription availability - Fast acting, long-term relief - Taken once or twice daily - 1st generation exhibits interpatient variability and adverse drug interactivity
2. Antacids and Alginates Aluminum Hydroxide Magaldrate Hydrotalcite	- Antacids raise pH of stomach/esophagus - Alginates block acid from reaching esophagus - Local - OTC availability - Fast acting, short-term relief - Frequent dosing necessary - Not useful in healing erosive esophagitis - Lack major side effects
3. Prokinetics Metoclopramide Domperidone Cisapride ATI-7505	- Block dopaminergic receptors and/or serotonin ($5\text{-}HT_4$) receptors - Increases esophageal peristalsis - Systemic - Prescription availability only - Slow acting, short-term relief - Taken twice daily - Large number of side effects
4. Histamine H_2-Receptor Antagonists (H_2RAs) Ranitidine Famotidine Cimetidine Nizatidine	- Reversibly block histamine H_2 receptors - Systemic - OTC and prescription availability - Slow acting, short-term relief - Tolerance developed within 1-2 weeks - No mucosal healing in cases of esophagitis
5. Potassium Competitive Acid Blockers (P CABs) Revaprazan Sorprazan AZD0865 PF-03716556	- Reversibly bind to K^+ binding region of H^+/K^+-ATPase - Systemic - Prescription availability only - Fast acting, long-term relief - No tolerance developed
6. Anti-Gastrin Agents Cholecystokinin$_2$ (CCK$_2$) receptor antagonists Anti-gastrin Vaccine (G-17DT)	- CCK$_2$ antagonists block CCK$_2$ receptors - Vaccine promotes antibody formation against gastrin 17 and glycine-extended G-17 - Systemic - Not yet commercially available - CCK$_2$ agents ineffective unless combined with PPIs - Gastrin vaccine recently discontinued

Anti-Gastrin Vaccine

Initial results investigating the antisecretory effect of G-17DT (Insegia™, previously known as Gastrimmune™), an anti-gastrin vaccine, have been very promising. G-17DT promotes antibody formation against both the amino acid gastrin 17 (G-17) and its precursor glycine-extended G-17; the former stimulates both acid secretion and lower esophageal sphincter function, while the latter is known to promote the growth of gastric tumors [67]. Pre-clinical animal models found that the vaccine was highly effective in blocking acid secretion, suggesting its potential use in treating GERD [68,69]. Furthermore, G-17DT showed efficacy against pancreatic tumors in Phase III clinical studies and gastric tumors in Phase II clinical studies [70]. Despite these promising results, the development of this vaccine was stopped in 2006 when the manufacturer filed for bankruptcy [35].

4. LONG-TERM EFFECTS OF PPI USE IN HUMANS

PPIs are the most commonly prescribed treatment option for GERD sufferers. While they have been found to be an appropriate short-term solution for assisting in the healing of esophagitis, as mentioned above relapse is common. There are believed to be two principal causes for this occurrence: 1) rebound acid hypersecretion is common upon withdrawal of PPI use and 2) the current generation of medications are unable to adequately address underlying pathophysiological changes, such as a lack of sufficient esophageal clearance [33]. Consequently, practitioners often continue treatment in patients even if presenting asymptomatic.

Continuous treatment raises a significant issue regarding the unknown long-term effects of treatment on indigenous microbiota colonies within the patient. It is well known that the normally low pH of the intragastric environment has a prophylactic impact against both the introduction of unwanted microorganisms and/or an over abundance of commensally beneficial biological populations. The introduction of PPIs can lead to sharp increases in the pH level of gastric acid. This increase in pH can in turn severely compromise this defense mechanism [71]. For example, *Clostridium difficile* is a bacterium commonly found in the environment, but is more pervasive in hospitals and nursing homes. Studies suggest patients using PPIs are at greater risk for developing infections resulting in nosocomial diarrhea

[72]. Further, it appears an increase in pH created through PPI use adversely impacts the inflammatory and immune response of the gastric mucosa. This has been supported by recent work showing PPI use in rats resulted in transcriptional changes in the apoptosis, inflammatory, immune, and stress responses of the gastric mucosa [73]. Additionally, earlier studies in rats also suggest PPIs increase mucosal thickness as well as ECL cell density, possibly leading to development of gastric tumors [74,75]. This body of prior work suggests PPI use may indeed cause a number of biological changes, the scope of which is not yet fully appreciated. Further understanding may be provided through additional studies on the long-term impact of PPI use.

The implications for altering the pH levels by PPI use may have far more reaching epidemiological consequences than currently understood. For example, changes in extracellular pH are known to alter intracellular pH. These changes can in turn impact the amount of internally-bound calcium ions [76,77], and as intracellular calcium levels are altered, changes in gene expression may result, potentially contributing to the growth of tumors [78-80]. There may be a causal link between long-term PPI use and undesired genetic alteration. The role extended PPI usage plays in this process has to be confirmed.

5. NON-GASTRIC ACID PRODUCTION

The overview of treatment options reviewed above focused on the gastric acid producing cells found in the stomach. Because the gastric proton pump pathways are prominent in this environment, emphasis is typically placed on PPIs and P-CABs for treatment. Each has been specifically configured to impact and regulate the gastric proton pump mechanism.

Significantly, a variety of recent studies have been conducted which indicate that H^+/K^+-ATPase enzyme pathways located in the stomach are also found elsewhere in the body. These sites include a number of acid-producing bacterial species within both the upper gastrointestinal tract and oral cavity. (We discuss these bacterial species further in Sections 7 and 8.) This important work has implications for clarifying the causes of GERD and the impact long-term PPI use has on the body. The causal relationship between long-term PPI use and GERD may be a function of: 1) these bacteria produce additional acid contributing to the onset of GERD, 2) PPI drugs are impacting areas outside of the stomach generating unwanted side effects, and/or 3) various microbiota populations may actually play contributing roles in the observed side effects associated with long-term therapy.

Non-Gastric H$^+$-ATPases

The gastric H$^+$/K$^+$-ATPase is a member of the P-type (ion-motive-phosphorylating) ATPase molecular family. There are also well known non-gastric members of this family, such as the H$^+$/K$^+$-ATPases and Na$^+$/K$^+$-ATPase enzymes found in muscle and nerve cells. These non-gastric counterparts are similar in structure to the gastric ATPases with an α and β subunit. The α component has a catalytic functional site, and the β subunit stabilizes the molecular structure of this heterodimer [15,16]. While the complete behavior pattern of these molecules remains unconfirmed, it is suggested that non-gastric H$^+$/K$^+$-ATPases are involved in maintaining K$^+$ homeostasis in K$^+$- and Na$^+$-scarce environments [16].

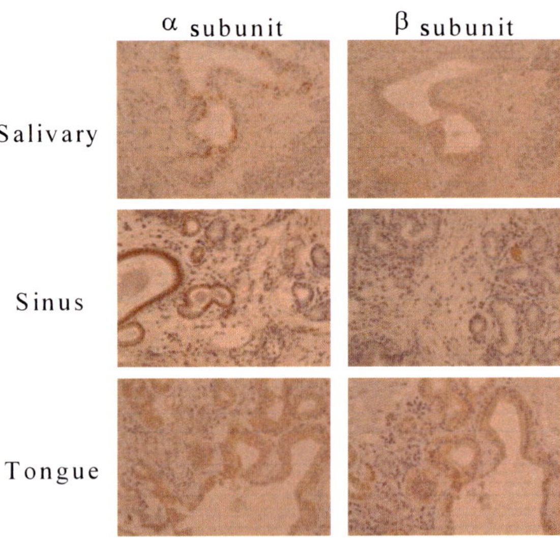

Figure 12. Immunohistochemical staining of proton pump subunits (α, left, and β, right) in human salivary gland, sinus, and tongue mucosa. Positive immunohistochemical staining is brown. Images shown at 20x original magnification. Reproduced with permission [13]. Copyright 2008 Wiley-VCH Verlag GmbH & Co. KGaA, Weinheim.

Immunohistochemical staining techniques used in our laboratory have verified the existence of both α and β subunits of H^+/K^+-ATPase in human tissues of the larynx [18,19] as well as lung [17]. Furthermore, H^+ ion-exchange pumps have also been confirmed in rat colon [81], rat kidney [82], rat and cockroach salivary glands [83-85], rabbit and human esophagus [86,87], and human lung cells [88]. Recent work in our laboratory has further shown that H^+/K^+-ATPases are expressed in human tongue, sinus, and salivary gland tissues (Figure 12).

Results from preliminary studies involving these non-gastric H^+/K^+-ATPases indicate the molecules likely play a key role in the therapy of GERD. As an example, studies performed with rat submandibular gland indicate that a disruption in acid-base equilibrium led to an adaptive change of the enzyme, specifically producing an 'activated state' of H^+/K^+-ATPase upon metabolic acidosis [83]. This provides a possible explanation as to how Na^+/H^+ antiport of the human esophagus might serve as a defense against high levels of acid, especially when refluxed from the stomach [86]. Further studies are needed to confirm initial results suggesting that non-gastric H^+/K^+-ATPases may act as direct sites for PPI and potassium-competitive acid blocker pharmacotherapy.

6. COMPARISON OF ATPASES WITHIN HUMANS, BACTERIA AND FUNGI

As mentioned above, PPIs are specifically designed to target the gastric acid pump H^+/K^+-ATPase enzyme. There are three ion-motive ATPase family types: 1) P-type or ion-motive-phosphorylating, 2) V-type or vacuolated, and 3) F-type or F_1F_0 ATPases [89]. The pathway for ion transport for P-type proton pumps is accomplished by coupling to a cycle of phosphorylation and dephosphorylation. P-type ATPases are not restricted exclusively to gastric proton pumps in humans. There are indeed a number of non-gastric varieties present including H^+/K^+-ATPases, Na^+/K^+-ATPases, and Ca^{2+}-ATPases, all of which fall into the P-type family [13,15,90].

Significantly, ion-motive ATPases are also located in both a variety of bacteria and fungi species. Bacteria are known to have both F-type ATPases [91] and P-Type ATPase enzymes. These have been found in a number of naturally occurring bacteria species including *Helicobacter pylori* and *Streptococcus pneumoniae* [92,93]. In fungi, the evidence is equally robust.

There are a variety of fungi found to contain P-type ATPase enzymes (H^+-ATPases) within the plasma membrane: *Candida albicans, Saccharomyces cerevisae, Cryptococcus neoformans, Pneumocystis carinii*, and *Asperigillus niger* [94,95]. Numerous studies strongly indicate there is a high homology among the various P-type ATPase enzymes [96-98], along with evidence for molecular mimicry between *H. pylori* and the H^+/K^+-ATPase of the parietal cells during development of autoimmune gastritis [99,100]. There is an abundance of evidence to support the existence of different bacteria and fungi resident populations which contain ion-motive ATPases within humans. Further studies are needed to confirm or deny the role these enzymes may have in PPI therapy [13,101].

7. ACID-PRODUCING BACTERIA AND FUNGI IN HUMANS

It was long believed that bacteria couldn't survive either the harsh acidic environment in the human stomach or esophagus. Not until 1980, upon the discovery of *H. pylori* in the stomach, did thinking change. More recent studies have confirmed bacteria are also found in the upper gastrointestinal tract [102]. Examples include strains of *Streptococcus* and *Lactobacilli*, which are themselves acid-producing and can also be found in the oral cavity and gastrointestinal tract [103]. Some of these bacteria are indigenous microbiota populations within the body, while others are introduced through food intake, such as fermented foods and dairy products. Similarly, fungi containing H^+-ATPases are known to naturally inhibit the human body.

The degree to which these acid-producing bacteria and fungi affect the development and progression of GERD is currently not known [104]. The possibility exists that the acid-producing species present in the esophagus and oral cavity may be contributing to the onset of GERD through the direct production of acid. Equally possible is that GERD drug therapy, specifically PPIs, may be inadvertently targeting the proton pumps of the commensal bacteria and fungi as extrinsic sites of action, resulting in adverse effects for the human microbiota. These ideas are supported by two observations: 1) the comparable structures of human and bacterial proton pumps, as described above, and 2) the mechanism to shut down the pumps is equivalent [13].

8. PPIs AND BACTERIA

In this section we summarize what is currently known about the effects that PPIs have on bacteria, particularly *H. pylori* and *C. difficile*. Section 9 follows with a discussion of PPI-fungi interactions.

Helicobacter Pylori

As discussed above, *H. pylori* is found in the stomach and has been studied extensively. The bacteria can progressively cause inflammation of the gastric mucosa, infection, and in severe instances, destruction of the gastric mucosa. This in turn may lead to stomach atrophy and/or cause intestinal metaplasia to develop. These conditions lead to reduced acid secretion and the proliferation of fecal-type organisms, which in turn overwhelm and drive out normally occurring *H. pylori* colonies [105]. This progression of events results in the stomach being far more susceptible to gastric cancer, as evidenced by higher incidence of gastric cancer in *H. pylori*-positive patients [106].

Clearly *H. pylori* can significantly impact not only gastric acid secretion, but the overall functionality of the stomach. Not surprisingly, this has resulted in efforts directed toward determining the underlying mechanism of how *H. pylori* infections impact patients with GERD [105,107-109]. Recent studies show a large increase in the occurrence of GERD within general populations, with a corresponding decrease in *H. pylori* infections. This leads to speculation about the bacterium possibly having a prophylactic role against GERD onset in patients [105,109,110]. Currently, there is insufficient evidence available to validate a causal relationship, despite recent studies which have attempted to identify such a link. Studies to date have been too small in scope and all have been epidemiological in nature [105,107-110].

The most common treatment regimes for therapy against *H. pylori* infections uses what has come to be known as "inhibitor-based triple therapies," the concurrent use of two antibiotics (amoxicillin and clarithromycin) along with one PPI [111]. The PPI is used because it raises the pH level of the stomach, allowing the antibiotics to be more effective against *H. pylori* infections [112]. However, an increase in resistance to antibiotics has been observed, raising doubts about the future efficacy of triple therapy approaches [113]. One recent method being tried to counteract the antibiotic resistance is "sequential therapy" which introduces the two antibodies sequentially, rather than concurrently. While early results of the sequential therapy technique are promising, further studies need to be carried out on larger populations to confirm its effectiveness [114].

For inhibitor-based triple therapies being carried out in patients that are both *H. pylori*-positive and symptomatic of GERD, it is typical to treat the *H. pylori* infection first [115]. But others argue that since *H. pylori*-negative GERD patients are usually found to have a slower initial response to PPI therapy, the PPI should be prescribed alone first [86]. Some experts support the view that a triple-based therapy does not adversely affect GERD or the efficacy of PPI use [116]. Given that the combination of the bacteria and PPI use raise the pH, others have argued that non-*H. pylori* bacteria are able to flourish in the higher pH environment [117,118]. The greater presence of these non-*H. pylori* colonies may increase infection and/or lead to the onset of atrophic gastritis and gastric cancer [119,120].

Early research in this area focused on the impact of three PPIs on *H. pylori*: lanosprazole, omeprazole, and pantoprazole—each of which was found to have a bacteriostatic effect on *H. pylori* [121,122]. Lansoprazole was determined to be the most effective drug through its suppression of the P-Type ATPase of the *H. pylori* [121]. Two more recent studies have further confirmed a direct link between PPIs and *H. pylori*. The first involved autoradiographic experiments which confirmed the existence of ^{3}H-lansoprazole uptake sites located near the plasma membrane of *H. pylori* [90]; the second showed that raboprazole directly suppresses *H. pylori* growth *in vivo* in gerbils [123].

Further studies involving lansoprazole, omeprazole, and pantoprazole suggested that each of the three PPIs was capable of suppressing the urease activity of *H. pylori* [124,125]. Contradictory evidence from later work draws into question whether lansoprazole was actually responsible for urease inhibition [126,127]. Further, there is still some question regarding the mechanism for suppression, since both independent and dependent pathways have been discussed [124,128,129]. Understanding the effect of PPIs on the urease enzyme pathway would identify a potential therapeutic target for the regulation and/or elimination of *H. pylori* infections [130]. The uncertainties surrounding the role of PPIs on *H. pylori* function suggest a great need for further research in this important area.

Clostridium Difficile

Extensive studies have also been conducted on another commonly occurring bacterium, *Clostridium difficile*. Most infections originate in a hospital setting after antibiotics have been administered, or alternately through poor sanitary conditions within the community [131,132]. *C. difficile* infections are known to cause diarrhea and, in more severe cases, pseudomembranous colitis and colonic perforation [133,134]. Initial entry into the body occurs through the oral cavity. If the strain is sufficiently resistant to the low pH level within the stomach, it can progress through the gastrointestinal tract and colonize in the colon. Once in the colon, the bacteria produce two toxins: A and B, both of which contribute to the pathogenesis of the disease [135]. Treatment is usually accomplished through use of anticlostridial antibiotics such as metronidazole or vancomycin; in non-responsive or severe cases, a total colectomy may be necessary [136,137].

Because gastric acid is the primary line of defense against *C. difficile*, it is important to understand the effect that the PPIs have on the bacterium. Similar to *H. pylori*, there are varying opinions regarding the impact of PPI treatments on *C. difficile*. Since PPI use leads to an increase in the pH level within the stomach and decreases gastric acid production, it has been argued that the PPI-induced environment is favorable for *C. difficile* growth. Some experts also believe that use of antibiotics negatively impacts other resident intestinal bacteria, in turn enabling large *C. difficile* colonies to grow opportunistically [138]. Some studies go so far as to speculate that PPI therapy is actually a stand alone cause for concern for increased risk of *C. difficile* infection [135,139,140]. But, based on results from epidemiological studies, others contend there isn't sufficient evidence to support a causal relationship given the complexity of the environments and the inability to adequately control for external causes [131,141,142]. Unlike *H. pylori*, *C. difficile* does not contain proton pumps, therefore any impact from PPIs is believed to be a result of an indirect mechanism.

It is readily acknowledged that there are enormous numbers of prescriptions being written and excessive use of PPIs by patients. A variety of studies confirm this as being a worldwide phenomenon. For example, one UK study found that, of 138 patients admitted with *C. difficile* infections, 63.7% were taking PPIs, while guidelines set by the National Institute for Clinical Excellence indicated there should have been only 39.8% on medication [143].

Other work done in Ireland [144], Australia [145], Canada [146], France [147], and the United States [148] also supported the UK study findings. Should a causal relationship between PPI use and *C. difficile* infections be confirmed, this over-prescription and use of PPIs will only exacerbate the number of infections already observed. Even if such a link is ultimately not confirmed, the increased health risks associated with long-term PPI usage is justification alone for more stringent international guidelines for drug dispensing and use.

Other Bacteria

Studies investigating PPI interaction with bacteria other than *H. pylori* and *C. difficile* have to date been limited. However, the results of one study indicated that long-term PPI use may increase the risk of cancers of the stomach and gatroesophageal junction [149]. This was evidenced by a correlation between bacterial-induced acetaldehyde production and hypochlorhydria, a side effect occasionally manifested during PPI therapy. The hypochlorhydria initiated by PPI use resulted in the overgrowth of aerobic bacteria within the stomach and led to carcinogenic levels of microbially-mediated acetaldehyde production from ethanol [149].

Most microbiota are prevented access to the upper aerodigestive tract by the usually low pH level within the environment. As PPI use continues over time within a patient, the gastric and upper aerodigestive pH levels rise, which can in turn permit the growth of opportunistic populations of microbiota such as β-hemolytic *Streptococcus*, a bacteria known to cause pneumonia, thereby increasing susceptibility to infectious diseases [150,151]. This has been supported by a 2006 study which showed gastric acid inhibitors caused an increase in risk among children for community-acquired pneumonia and acute gastroenteritis [27]. Also evident was an increase in the incidence of intestinal and respiratory infection believed to be caused by the inhibitory effect of gastric acid inhibitors on leukocyte function, which in turn compromises the immune system. Gastric acid inhibition was also believed to be potentially responsible for increased risk of infection due to an abnormal microbiota environment [151].

There is additional work indicating that the growth of commensal bacterial found outside of the stomach may be impacted by PPIs [101].

Specifically, acid-producing bacteria such as *Streptococci* and *Lactobacilli*, which are present in both the oral cavity and gastrointestinal tract [102,151,152], might contain secondary reactive sites for PPIs [13]. Additionally, because PPI treatment occurs via a systemic delivery mechanism, the drugs can significantly impact non-parietal bacteria, targeting the proton pumps found in those bacteria, given their similarities in proton pump structure relative to human H^+/K^+-ATPases. Finally, these acid-producing bacteria may also be generating additional acid within the esophagus and oral cavity, thereby accelerating the onset of GERD [13].

As discussed in one of our recent publications, we found both morphological changes and inhibition of growth taking place for a variety of *Lactobacilli* strains when exposed to supra-physiological doses of pantoprazole [101]. We believe that these *in vivo* changes can be linked to: 1) direct inhibition of normal bacteria growth resulting from PPI use, and 2) PPIs indirectly impacting the oral and gastrointestinal microenvironments by increasing the pH. While these results suggest that lansoprazole is inadvertently affecting commensal bacteria in humans, further research is needed to explore the mechanisms by which bacteria are affected by PPIs.

9. PPIs and Fungi

The presence of a variety of fungal species within the human body is well known. Typically these are acquired either commensally or opportunistically. It is also well known that these fungi possess H^+-ATPases which, like the bacterial proton pumps, may be impacted by PPI therapy. A number of *in vitro* studies demonstrate that the PPIs possess antifungal properties. For example, treating *C. albicans* and *S. cerevisiae* with omeprazole resulted in pH-dependent growth inhibition of both species, and the PPI lansoprazole was also found to inhibit *C. albicans* growth [153]. In another study, the growth of several fungi—including *Candida*, *Saccharomyces*, and *Aspergillus*—was inhibited by a novel styryl ketone designed to target H^+-ATPase [154]. To date, *in vivo* studies of PPI-fungi interactions have not yet been carried out, suggesting an area of potential future research.

10. CONCLUSION

In summary, while gastroesophageal reflux disease is a commonly diagnosed disease, the use of proton pump inhibitors as the main form of treatment deserves more careful consideration. Research to date has suggested that the PPIs may be also targeting the proton pumps of naturally occurring bacteria and fungi present within the human body, disturbing the natural human flora. Because expression of the proton pump has been identified in non-gastric tissue, the effects of proton pump inhibitors may have far greater implications than previously thought. There may be both short-term, micropharmacological therapeutic implications and long-term epidemiological consequences yet to be fully realized. Further research is needed to gain a more complete understanding of the impact PPIs have on the natural human microbiota.

REFERENCES

[1]   Ferguson, D. D. *Expert Opin. Pharmacother.* 2007, 8, 39-47.
[2]   Tutuian, R. *J. Gastrointestin. Liver Dis.* 2006, 15, 243-247.
[3]   Locke III, G. R. *Gastroenterol. Clin. North Am.* 1996, 25, 1-19.
[4]   Locke III, G. R.; Talley, N. H.; Fett, S. L.; Zinsmeister, A. R.; Melton, L. J. *Gastroenterology* 1997, 112, 1448-1456.
[5]   Altman, K. W.; Stephens, R. M.; Lyttle, C. S.; Weiss, K. B. *Laryngoscope* 2005, 115, 1145-1153.
[6]   Fass, R. *J. Clin. Gastroenterol.* 2007, 41, 131-137.
[7]   Lagergren, J. *Best Pract. Res. Clin. Gastroenterol.* 2006, 20, 803-812.
[8]   Baker, D. E. *Rev. Gastroenterol. Disord.* 2006, 6, 22-34.
[9]   Slattery, E.; Theyventhiran, R.; Cullen, G.; Kennedy, F.; Ridge, C.; Nolan, K.; Kidney, R.; O'Donoghue, D. P.; Mulcahy, H. E. *Eur. J. Gastroenterol. Hepatol.* 2007, 19, 461-464.
[10]   Falk, G. W. *Clev. Clin. J. Med.* 2001, 68, 415-424.
[11]   Anderson, L. A.; Watson, R. G.; Murphy, S. J.; Johnston, B. T.; Comber, H.; McGuigan, J.; Reynolds, J. V.; Murray, L. J. *World J. Gastroenterol.* 2007, 13, 1585-1594.
[12]   Bujanda, L. *Am. J. Gastroenterol.* 2000, 95, 3374-3382.

[13] Vesper, B. J.; Altman, K. W.; Elseth, K. M.; Haines III, G. K.; Pavlova, S. I.; Tao, L.; Tarjan, G.; Radosevich, J. A. *ChemMedChem* 2008, 3, 552-559.

[14] Vesper, B. J.; Jawdi, A.; Altman, K. W.; Haines III, G. K.; Tao, L.; Radosevich, J. A. *Curr. Drug Metab.* 2009, 10, 84-89.

[15] Jaisser, F.; Beggah, A. T. *Am. J. Physiol.* 1999, 276, F812-F824.

[16] Crambert, G.; Horisberger, J. D.; Modyanov, N. N.; Geering, K. *Am. J. Physiol. Cell Physiol.* 2002, 283, C305-C314.

[17] Altman, K. W.; Waltonen, J. D.; Tarjan, G.; Radosevich, J. A.; Haines III, G. K. *Ann. Otol. Rhinol. Laryngol.* 2007, 116, 229-234.

[18] Altman, K. W.; Waltonen, J. D.; Hammer, N. D.; Radosevich, J. A.; Haines III, G. K. *Otolaryngol. Head Neck Surg.* 2005, 133, 718-724.

[19] Altman, K. W.; Haines III, G. K.; Hammer, N. D.; Radosevich, J. A. *Laryngoscope* 2003, 113, 1927-1930.

[20] Cui, G.; Waldum, H. L. *World J. Gastroenterol.* 2007, 13, 493-496.

[21] Hou, W.; Schubert, M. L. *Curr. Opin. Gastroenterol.* 2006, 22, 593-598.

[22] Sachs, G.; Shin, J. M.; Briving, C.; Wallmark, B.; Hersey, S. *Annu. Rev. Pharmacol. Toxicol.* 1995, 35, 277-305.

[23] Schubert, M. L. *Curr. Opin. Gastroenterol.* 2005, 21, 636-643.

[24] Scarpignato, C.; Pelosini, I.; Di Mario, F. *Dig. Dis.* 2006, 24, 11-46.

[25] Black, J.; Kalindjian, S. *Pharmacol. Toxicol.* 2002, 91, 275-281.

[26] Andersson, K.; Carlsson, E. *Pharmacol. Therapeut.* 2005, 108, 294-307.

[27] Geibel, J. P.; Wagner, C. A. *Rev. Physiol. Biochem. Pharmacol.* 2006, 156, 45-60.

[28] Pettit, M. *Pharm. World Sci.* 2005, 27, 432-435.

[29] Chiba, N.; De Gara, C. J.; Wilkinson, J. M.; Hunt, R. H. *Gastroenterology* 1997, 112, 1798-1810.

[30] Huang, J. Q.; Hunt, R. H. *Best Pract. Res. Clin. Gastroenterol.* 2001, 15, 355-370.

[31] Metz, D. C.; Inadomi, J. M.; Howden, C. W.; Veldhuyzen van Zanten, S. J.; Bytzer, P. *Am. J. Gastroenterol.* 2007, 102, 642-653.

[32] Colin-Jones, D. G. *Aliment. Pharmacol. Ther.* 1995, 9, 9-14.

[33] Pohle, T.; Domschke, W. *Langenbecks Arch. Surg.* 2000, 385, 317-323.

[34] Sachs, G. *Pharmacotherapy* 2003, 23, 68S-73S.

[35] Vakil, N. *Rev. Gastroenterol. Disord.* 2008, 8, 117-122.

[36] Der, G. *Gastroenterol. Nurs.* 2003, 26, 182-190.

[37] *Nursing* 2002, 32, 18, 20.

[38] Kollmeier, A. P.; Eddleston, J.; Zuraw, B. L.; Christiansen, S. C. *J. Allergy Clin. Immunol.* 2004, 114, 975-977.

[39] van Zyl, J.; van Rensburg, C.; Vieweg, W.; Fischer, R. *Digestion* 2004, 70, 61-69.

[40] Jensen, R. T. *Basic Clin. Pharmacol. Toxicol.* 2006, 98, 4-19.

[41] Hetzel, D. J.; Dent, J.; Reed, W. D.; Narielvala, F. M.; Mackinnon, M.; McCarthy, J. H.; Mitchell, B.; Beveridge, B. R.; Laurence, B. H.; Gibson, G. G. *Gastroenterology* 1988, 95, 903-912.

[42] Cundy, T.; Dissanayake, A. *Clin. Endocrinol.* 2008, 69, 338-341.

[43] Wright, M. J.; Proctor, D. D.; Insogna, K. L.; Kerstetter, J. E. *Nutr. Rev.* 2008, 66, 103-108.

[44] Tonini, M.; Giorgio, R. D.; Ponti, F. D. *Expert Opin. Ther. Pat.* 2003, 13, 639-649.

[45] Vakily, M.; Zhang, W.; Wu, J.; Atkinson, S. N.; Mulford, D. *Curr. Med. Res. Opin.* 2009, 25, 627-638.

[46] Metz, D. C.; Howden, C. W.; Perez, M. C.; Larsen, L. M.; O'Neil, J. M. *Gastroenterology* 2008, 134, A-171.

[47] Kwon, D.; Chae, J. B.; Park, C. W.; Kim, Y. S.; Lee, S. M.; Kim, E. J.; Huh, I. H.; Kim, D. Y.; Cho, K. D. *Arznei.-Forschung* 2001, 51, 204-213.

[48] Periclou, A. P.; Goldwater, R.; Lee, S. M.; Park, D. W.; Kim, D. Y.; Cho, K. D.; Boileau, F.; Jung, W. T. *Clin. Pharmacol. Ther.* 2000, 68, 304-311.

[49] Negma-Lerads. (2001). Tenatoprazole (TU-199) Investigator's Brochure.

[50] Domagala, F.; Ficheux, H.; Houin, G.; Barre, J. *Arznei.-Forschung* 2006, 56, 33-39.

[51] Galmiche, J. P.; Sacher-Huvelin, S.; Bruley des Varannes, S.; Vavasseur, F.; Taccoen, A.; Fiorentini, P.; Homerin, M. *Aliment Pharmacol. Ther.* 2005, 21, 575-582.

[52] Hibbs, A. M.; Lorch, S. A. *Pediatrics* 2006, 118, 746-752.

[53] Sanger, G. J.; Alpers, D. H. *Neurogastroenterol. Motil.* 2008, 20, 177-184.

[54] Reddymasu, S. C.; Soykan, I.; McCallum, R. W. *Am. J. Gastroenterol.* 2007, 102, 2036-2045.

[55] Robinson, P. *Am. J. Gastroenterol.* 2008, 103, 1049.

[56] Camilleri, M.; Vazquez-Roque, M. I.; Burton, D.; Ford, T.; McKinzie, S.; Zinsmeister, A. R.; Druzgala, P. *Neurogastroenterol. Motil.* 2007, 19, 30-38.

[57] ARYx Therapeutics, Inc. (2008). ARYx Therapeutics, Inc. Announces Successful Results of QT study on ATI-7505. http://www.drugs.com/clinical_trials/aryx-therapeutics-inc-announces-successful-results-qt-study-ati-7505-4997.html. Accessed March 5, 2009.

[58] Geibel, J. P. *World J. Gastroenterol.* 2005, 11, 5259-5265.

[59] Mori, H.; Tonai-Kachi, H.; Ochi, Y.; Taniguchi, Y.; Ohshiro, H.; Takahashi, N.; Aihara, T.; Hirao, A.; Kato, T.; Sakakibara, M.; Kurebayashi, Y. *J. Pharmacol. Exp. Ther.* 2009, 328, 671-679.

[60] Kidd, M.; Modlin, I. M.; Tang, L. H. *Dig. Surg.* 1998, 15, 209-217.

[61] Wank, S. A. *Am. J. Gastroenterol.* 1998, 274, G607-G613.

[62] Makovec, F.; Revel, L.; Letari, O.; Mennuni, L.; Impicciatore, M. *Eur. J. Pharmacol.* 1999, 369, 81-90.

[63] Beglinger, C.; Degen, L.; Schroller, S.; D'Amato, M.; Persiani, S. *Gut* 2005, 54, A36.

[64] Morita, H.; Miura, N.; Hori, Y.; Matsunaga, Y.; Ukawa, H.; Suda, H.; Yoneta, T.; Kurimoto, T.; Itoh, Z. *Gastroenterology* 2001, 120, A331.

[65] Reubi, J. C.; Schaer, J. C.; Waser, B. *Cancer Res.* 1997, 57, 1377-1386.

[66] [66] Grabowska, A. M.; Morris, T. M.; McKenzie, A. J.; Kumari, R.; Hamano, H.; Emori, Y.; Yoshinaga, K.; Watson, S. A. *Regul. Pept.* 2008, 146, 46-57.

[67] Iwase, K.; Evers, B. M.; Hellmich, M. R.; Guo, Y. S.; Higashide, S.; Kim, H. J.; Townsend Jr., C. M. *Gastroenterology* 1997, 113, 782-790.

[68] Smith, A. M.; Morris, T.; Justin, T.; Michaeli, D.; Watson, S. A. *Aliment. Pharmacol. Ther.* 2001, 15, 1981-1988.

[69] Justin, T.; Watson, S.; Michaeli, D.; Hardcastle, J.; Steele, R. *Gastroenterology* 1995, 108, A125.

[70] Gilliam, A. D.; Watson, S. A. *Expert Opin. Biol. Ther.* 2007, 7, 397-404.

[71] Nwokolo, C. U.; Loft, D. E.; Holder, R.; Langman, M. J. S. *Eur. J. Gastroenterol. Hepatol.* 1994, 6, 697-699.

[72] Dial, S.; Delaney, J. A. C.; Barkun, A. N.; Suissa, S. *JAMA* 2005, 294, 2989-2995.

[73] Norsett, K. G.; Laegreid, A.; Langaas, M.; Worlund, S.; Rossmark, R.; Waldum, H. L.; Sandvik, A. K. *Physiol. Genomics* 2005, 22, 24-32.

[74]   Havu, N. *Digestion* 1986, 35, 42-55.

[75]   Ekman, L.; Hansson, E.; Havu, N.; Carlsson, E.; Lundberg, C. *Scand. J. Gastroenterol. Suppl.* 1985, 108, 53-69.

[76]   Taggart, M.; Austin, C.; Wray, S. *J. Physiol.* 1994, 475, 285-292.

[77]   Tolkovsky, A. M.; Richards, C. D. *Neuroscience* 1987, 22,

[78]   Saito, K.; Uzawa, K.; Endo, Y.; Kato, Y.; Nakashima, D.; Ogawara, K.; Shiiba, M.; Bukawa, H.; Yokoe, H.; Tanzawa, H. *Oncol. Rep.* 2006, 15, 49-55.

[79]   Endo, Y.; Uzawa, K.; Mochida, Y.; Shiiba, M.; Bukawa, H.; Yokoe, H.; Tanzawa, H. *Int. J. Cancer* 2004, 110, 225-231.

[80]   Chung, F. Y.; Lin, S. R.; Lu, C. Y.; Yeh, C. S.; Chen, F. M.; Hsieh, J. S.; Huang, T. J.; Wang, J. Y. *Am. J. Surg. Pathol.* 2006, 30, 969-974.

[81]   Lee, J. S.; Rajendran, V. M.; Mann, A. S.; Kashgarian, M.; Binder, H. J. *J. Clin. Invest.* 1995, 96, 2002-2008.

[82]   Sangan, P.; Rajendran, V. M.; Mann, A. S.; Kashgarian, M.; Binder, H. J. *Am. J. Physiol. Cell Physiol.* 1997, 272, C685-C696.

[83]   Roussa, E.; Thevenod, F.; Sabolic, I. *J. Histochem. Cytochem.* 1998, 46, 91-100.

[84]   Roussa, E.; Thevenod, F. *Eur. J. Morphol.* 1998, 36(suppl), 147-152.

[85]   Just, F.; Walz, B. *Cell Tissue Res.* 1994, 278, 161-170.

[86]   Tobey, N. A.; Koves, G.; Orlando, R. C. *Am. J. Gastroenterol.* 1998, 93, 2075-2081.

[87]   Layden, T. J.; Agnone, L. M.; Schmidt, L. N.; Hakim, B.; Goldstein, J. L. *Gastroenterology* 1990, 99, 909-917.

[88]   Fischer, H.; Widdicombe, J. H.; Illek, B. *Am. J. Physiol. Cell Physiol.* 2002, 282, C736-C743.

[89]   McCarty, R. E. *J. Exp. Biol.* 1992, 172, 431-441.

[90]   Nakamura, M.; Matsui, H.; Serizawa, H.; Tsuchimoto, K. *J. Clin. Biochem. Nutr.* 2007, 41, 154-159.

[91]   Magalhaes, P. P.; Paulino, T. P.; Thedei Jr., G.; Ciancaglini, P. *Comp. Biochem. Physiol. B Biochem. Mol. Biol.* 2005, 140, 589-597.

[92]   Melchers, K.; Herrmann, L.; Mauch, F.; Bayle, D.; Heuermann, D.; Weitzenegger, T.; Schuhmacher, A.; Sachs, G.; Haas, R.; Bode, G.; Bensch, K.; Schafer, K. P. *Acta Physiol. Scand. Suppl.* 1998, 643, 123-125.

[93]   Hoskins, J.; Alborn, W. E.; Arnold, J. *J. Bacteriol.* 2001, 183, 5709-5717.

[94] Afeltra, J.; Verweij, P. E. *Eur. J. Clin. Microbiol. Infect. Dis.* 2003, 22, 397-407.

[95] Perlin, D. S.; Seto-Young, D.; Monk, B. C. *Ann. NY Acad. Sci.* 1997, 834, 609-617.

[96] Magalhaes, P. P.; Paulino, T. P.; Thedei Jr., G.; Larson, R. E.; Ciancaglini, P. *Arch. Oral Biol.* 2003, 48, 815-824.

[97] Kuhlbrandt, W. *Nat. Rev. Mol. Cell Biol.* 2004, 5, 282-295.

[98] Axelsen, K. B.; Palmgren, M. G. *Plant Physiol.* 2001, 126, 696-706.

[99] Amedei, A.; Bergman, M. P.; Appelmelk, B. J.; Azzurri, A.; Benagiano, M.; Tamburini, C.; van der Zee, R.; Telford, J. L.; Vandenbroucke-Grauls, C. M.; D'Elios, M. M.; Del Prete, G. *J. Exp. Med.* 2003, 198, 1147-1156.

[100] D'Elios, M. M.; Appelmelk, B. J.; Amedei, A.; Bergman, M. P.; Del Prete, G. *Trends Mol. Med.* 2004, 10, 316-323.

[101] Altman, K. W.; Chhaya, V.; Hammer, N. D.; Pavlova, S.; Vesper, B. J.; Tao, L.; Radosevich, J. A. *Laryngoscope* 2008, 118, 599-604.

[102] Pei, Z.; Bini, E.; Yang, L.; Zhou, M.; Francois, F.; Blaser, M. J. *Proc. Natl. Acad. Sci. USA* 2004, 101, 4250-4255.

[103] Kullen, M. J.; Klaenhammer, T. R. *Mol. Microbiol.* 1999, 33, 1152-1161.

[104] Pei, Z.; Yang, L.; Peek, J., R. M.; Levine, S. M.; Pride, D. T.; Blaser, M. J. *World J. Gastroenterol.* 2005, 11, 7277-7283.

[105] Axon, A. *J. Clin. Gastroenterol.* 2006, 40, 15-19.

[106] Uemura, N.; Okamoto, S.; Yamamoto, S.; Matsumura, N.; Yamaguchi, S.; Yamakido, M.; Taniyama, K.; Sasaki, N.; Schlemper, R. J. *N. Engl. J. Med.* 2001, 345, 784-789.

[107] Delaney, B.; McColl, K. *Aliment. Pharmacol. Ther.* 2005, 22, 32-40.

[108] Lai, L. H.; Sung, J. J. *Best Pract. Res. Clin. Gastroenterol* 2007, 21, 261-279.

[109] Thor, P. J.; Blaut, U. *J. Physiol. Pharmacol.* 2006, 57, 81-90.

[110] Moayyedi, P.; Talley, N. J. *Lancet* 2006, 367, 2086-2100.

[111] Pilotto, A.; Franceschi, M.; Rassu, M.; Leandro, G.; Bozzola, L.; Furlan, F.; Di Mario, F. *Dig. Liver Dis.* 2000, 32, 667-672.

[112] Gambaro, C.; Bilardi, C.; Dulbecco, P.; Iiritano, E.; Zentilin, P.; Mansia, C.; Usai, P.; Vigneri, S.; Savarino, V. *Dig. Liver Dis.* 2003, 35, 763-767.

[113] Bergamaschi, A.; Magrini, A.; Pietroiusti, A. *Recent Patents Anti-Infect. Drug Disc.* 2007, 2, 197-205.

[114] Vakil, N. *Am. J. Gastroenterol.* 2009, 104, 26-30.

[115] Parente, F. R.; Bargiggia, S. A.; Anderloni, A. *Scand. J. Gastroenterol.* 2006, 41, 1121-1125.

[116] Kuipers, E. J. *Basic Clin. Pharmacol. Toxicol.* 2006, 99, 187-194.

[117] Lee, J. M.; O'Morain, C. A. *Gut* 1998, 43, S14-S20.

[118] Williams, C.; McColl, K. E. *Aliment. Pharmacol. Ther.* 2006, 23, 3-10.

[119] Sanduleanu, S.; Jonkers, D.; De Bruine, A.; Hameeteman, W.; Stockbrugger, R. W. *Aliment. Pharmacol. Ther.* 2001, 15, 379-388.

[120] Sanduleanu, S.; Jonkers, D.; De Bruine, A.; Hameeteman, W.; Stockbrugger, R. W. *Dig. Liver Dis.* 2001, 33, 707-719.

[121] Mauch, F.; Bode, G.; Malfertheiner, P. *Am. J. Gastroenterol.* 1993, 88, 1801-1802.

[122] Megraud, F.; Boyanova, L.; Lamouliatte, H. *Lancet* 1991, 337, 1486.

[123] Suzuki, H.; Miyazawa, M.; Nagahashi, S.; Sato, M.; Bessho, M.; Nagata, H.; Miura, S.; Ishii, H. *J. Gastroenterol. Hepatol.* 2003, 18, 787-795.

[124] Tsuchiya, M.; Imamura, L.; Park, J. B.; Kobashi, K. *Biol. Pharm. Bull.* 1995, 18, 1053-1056.

[125] Bugnoli, M.; Bayeli, P. F.; Rappuoli, R.; Pennatini, C.; Figura, N.; Crabtree, J. E. *Eur. J. Gastroenterol. Hepatol.* 1993, 5, 683-686.

[126] Nagata, K.; Takagi, E.; Tsuda, M.; Nakazawa, T.; Satoh, H.; Nakao, M.; Okamura, H.; Tamura, T. *Antimicrob. Agents Chemother.* 1995, 39, 567-570.

[127] Nakao, M.; Tada, M.; Tsuchimori, K.; Uekata, M. *Eur. J. Clin. Microbiol. Infect. Dis.* 1995, 14, 391-399.

[128] McGowan, C. C.; Cover, T. L.; Blaser, M. J. *Gastroenterology* 1994, 107, 1573-1578.

[129] Kuhler, T. C.; Fryklund, J.; Bergman, N. A.; Weilitz, J.; Lee, A.; Larsson, H. *J. Med. Chem.* 1995, 38, 4906-4916.

[130] Scott, D. R.; Marcus, E. A.; Weeks, D. L.; Sachs, G. *Gastroenterology* 2002, 123, 187-195.

[131] Cunningham, R. *CMAJ* 2006, 175, 757.

[132] Wilcox, M. H.; Mooney, L.; Bendall, R.; Settle, C. D.; Fawley, W. N. *J. Antimicrob. Chemother.* 2008, 62, 388-396.

[133] Thomas, C.; Stevenson, M.; Riley, T. V. *J. Antimicrob. Chemother.* 2003, 51, 1339-1350.

[134] Halsey, J. *Am. J. Health Syst. Pharm.* 2008, 65, 705-715.

[135] Kaur, S.; Vaishnavi, C.; Prasad, K. K.; Ray, P.; Kochhar, R. *Microbiol. Immunol.* 2007, 51, 1209-1214.

[136] Gerding, D. N.; Muto, C. A.; Owens Jr., R. C. *Clin. Infect. Dis.* 2008, 46, S32-S42.

[137] Bartlett, J. G. *Clin. Infect. Dis.* 2008, 46, S4-S11.

[138] Kyne, L.; Hamel, M. B.; Polavaram, R.; Kelly, C. P. *Clin. Infect. Dis.* 2002, 34, 346-353.

[139] Yearsley, K. A.; Gilby, L. J.; Ramadas, A. V.; Kubiak, E. M.; Fone, D. L.; Allison, M. C. *Aliment. Pharmacol. Ther.* 2006, 24, 613-619.

[140] Dial, S.; Alrasadi, K.; Manoukian, C.; Huang, A.; Menzies, D. *CMAJ* 2004, 171, 33-38.

[141] Lowe, D. O.; Mamdani, M. M.; Kopp, A.; Low, D. E.; Juurlink, D. N. *Clin. Infect. Dis.* 2006, 43, 1272-1276.

[142] Louie, T. J.; Meddings, J. *CMAJ* 2004, 171, 45-46.

[143] Choudhry, M. N.; Soran, H.; Ziglam, H. M. *QJM* 2008, 101, 445-448.

[144] Sebastian, S. S.; Kernan, N.; Qasim, A.; O'Morain, C. A.; Buckley, M. *Ir. J. Med. Sci.* 2003, 172, 115-117.

[145] Naunton, M.; Peterson, G. M.; Bleasel, M. D. *J. Clin. Pharm. Ther.* 2000, 25, 333-340.

[146] McBride, J. E.; Pater, J. L.; Dorland, J. L.; Lam, Y. M. *Ann. Pharmacother.* 1997, 31, 411-416.

[147] Marie, I.; Moutot, A.; Tharrasse, A.; Hellot, M. F.; Robaday, S.; Herve, F.; Levesque, H. *Rev. Med. Interne* 2007, 28, 86-93.

[148] Brandhagen, D. J.; Pheley, A. M.; Onstad, G. R.; Freeman, M. L.; Lurie, N. *J. Gen. Intern. Med.* 1995, 10, 513-515.

[149] Vakevainen, S.; Tillonen, J.; Salaspuro, M.; Jousimies-Somer, H.; Nuutinen, H.; Farkkila, M. *Aliment. Pharmacol. Ther.* 2000, 14, 1511-1518.

[150] Simms, H. H.; De Maria, E.; McDonald, L.; Peterson, D.; Robinson, A.; Buchard, K. W. *J. Trauma* 1991, 31, 531-536.

[151] Canani, R. B.; Cirillo, P.; Roggero, P.; Romano, C.; Malamisura, B.; Terrin, G.; Passariello, A.; Manguso, F.; Morelli, L.; Guarino, A.; Working Group on Intestinal Infections of the Italian Society of Pediatric Gastroenterology Hepatology and Nutrition (SIGENP). *Pediatrics* 2006, 117, e817-e820.

[152] Koll, P.; Mandar, R.; Marcotte, H.; Leibur, E.; Mikelsaar, M.; Hammarstrom, L. *Oral Microbiol. Immunol.* 2008, 23, 139-147.

[153] Biswas, S. K.; Yokoyama, K.; Kamei, K.; Nishimura, K.; Miyaji, M. *Med. Mycol.* 2001, 39, 283-285.

[154] Manavathu, E. K.; Dimmock, J. R.; Vashishtha, S. C.; Chandrasekar, P. H. *Antimicrob. Agents Chemother.* 1999, 43, 2950-2959.

In: Reflux Disease: Causes, Symptoms and ...   ISBN: 978-1-61668-694-9
Editor: G. M. Esposito, pp. 73-96   © 2010 Nova Science Publishers, Inc.

Chapter III

AN UPDATE ON PEDIATRIC GASTROESOPHAGEAL REFLUX DISEASE

Sunny Zaheed Hussain[1],[*] and Vasundhara Tolia[2]
[1] WK Pediatric GI Specialists, Shreveport, LA, USA;
[2]Michigan State University, MI, USA.

ABSTRACT

Gastroesophageal reflux disease (GERD) is one of the most common disorders in the pediatric population. Regurgitation of gastric contents into the lower esophagus is a physiologic event termed gastroesophageal reflux (GER) and cause minimal symptoms. However, when frequent symptoms impair quality of life and/or cause complications, it is called GERD. Symptoms can vary at different ages and can also affect other systems such as respiratory, dental and otolarygological organs.

Over the last decade, a more scientific and evidence-based understanding in this area has helped the professionals better understand GERD in children. In this chapter, we briefly discuss the advances in pathophysiology, epidemiology, clinical presentation, diagnostic

---

[*] Correspondence concerning this article should be addressed to: Dr. Sunny Zaheed Hussain,M.D., WK Pediatric GI Specialists, Suite: 305, 1801 Fairfield Avenue Shreveport, LA 71104 Ph 318-629-7769. Fax 318-629-7768; Cell Text: 202-258-8595; Email: Shussain@wkhs.com

modalities and management of pediatric GERD. Emerging data on natural history of Pediatric GERD are also reviewed.

Gastroesophageal reflux disease (GERD), defined as a condition that develops when the reflux of stomach contents causes troublesome symptoms and/or complications, is a common disorder prevalent in many countries. Gastroesophageal reflux (GER) represents one of the most common conditions referred to a pediatric gastroenterologist for children of all ages [1]. The distinction between "physiologic" GER and "pathologic" GERD is important. Complicated GERD includes erosive esophagitis with or without bleeding, ulcerative esophagitis, and esophageal strictures. GERD is a well established risk factor for Barrett's esophagus (BE) and esophageal adenocarcinoma, the most rapidly rising cancer in the western world [1,2].

Gastroesophageal reflux is classified as follows:

Physiologic / functional GER: Most commonly seen in infants; nuisance symptoms with normal growth and development and no complications. No pharmacotherapy is needed.

GERD: Patients frequently experience complications affecting their quality of life, requiring careful evaluation and treatment.

Secondary GER/GERD: An underlying condition may predispose to gastroesophageal reflux; e.g.; developmental delay, cystic fibrosis, tracheo-esophageal fistula (TEF) with esophageal atresia, or gastric outlet obstruction.

PATHOPHYSIOLOGY

Previously, GER in infancy and childhood was thought to be due to decreased lower esophageal sphincter (LES) tone. Currently, the major mechanism has been demonstrated to be inappropriate transient LES relaxation (TLESR) [3]. Relative increase in intragastric liquid volume in conjunction with abdominal wall muscle contraction, and supine and "slumped" positioning in infancy also contribute to symptoms of GER, mainly regurgitation. In uncomplicated GER, delayed gastric emptying is rare, but may be a contributing factor is refractory cases.

The presence of a hiatal hernia may worsen GERD by displacing LES into the chest and reflux can be facilitated by the lower intrathoracic pressure [4]. This along with spasticity, recumbent position, straining for constipation and decreased salivation may further aggravate reflux in developmentally challenged children. Intractable GERD is commonly seen in children with mental retardation and cerebral palsy because of their neurogenic bowel [2].

Other lifestyle factors predisposing to GER include smoking, alcohol, poor dietary habits (e.g., overeating, eating late at night, assuming a supine position shortly after eating), certain foods (e.g., greasy, highly acidic), motility disorders and obesity. Obesity has been associated with an increase in the risk of GERD and its complications by imposing mechanical stresses on the esophagogastric junction by increased intragastric pressure and anatomic disruption of the esophagogastric junction [5]. Psychological stress may be another factor responsible for increasing GERD symptoms.

EPIDEMIOLOGY

Traditionally, GERD has been viewed as a disease of the western world and thought to be uncommon in the developing countries. It has been suggested that there is an increasing trend in the prevalence of GERD over the last two decades. Several multicultural issues exist in the epidemiology of GERD. Although the prevalence of GER in infancy appears to be highest in North America and Europe, epidemiologic data from the Indian subcontinent, Thailand and Indonesia are emerging [6]. Recognition of language barriers in understanding the common terms used to describe reflux symptoms should be kept in mind while evaluating patients with different ethnic backgrounds. Studying racial and geographic differences in GERD and its complications are important as they highlight environmental or genetic influences in etiology and increase our understanding of the disease pathogenesis and management.

This is best studied using questionnaires filled by children over eight years of age with the help of their caretakers, if needed. Gastroesophageal reflux disease symptom questionnaires have been developed and tested prospectively and shown to be useful in distinguishing infants and young children with symptomatic GERD from healthy children [7]. Several other studies have followed corroborating and validating the issues of questionnaires involving pediatric GERD [8,9].

Such questionnaires have also been successfully utilized in following the course of therapeutic trials to determine outcome. The prevalence of GER in infants has been studied in predominantly Caucasian suburban infants from US, Australia and Italy using detailed questionnaires. Gastroesophageal reflux is most commonly seen in infancy, with a peak at age 1-4 months. Approximately 85% of infants vomit during the first week of life, and 60-70% manifest clinical GER at age 3-4 months. GER/GERD can be seen in otherwise healthy children of all ages. Esophageal symptoms of GER are frequent in adolescents as shown in a study using a cross-sectional questionnaire administered to 14-18 year-old students at two high schools. Fewer than 25% of 1,286 participants with reflux symptoms consulted a physician and/or took medications [10].

The role of *Helicobacter pylori (H pylori)* in GERD remains controversial, particularly in children, because there are conflicting published data. Adult studies suggested that *H pylori* infection may protect against GERD by causing atrophic gastritis, which leads to reduced gastric acid secretion. In two prospective pediatric studies, eradication of *H pylori* was not associated with increased symptoms of GER in children and adolescents [11]. However, a more recent retrospective analysis of 420 pediatric patients indicated that there is a significantly higher prevalence of reflux esophagitis in an *H pylori*-infected cohort independent of age or sex; suggesting that *H pylori* infection in children is positively associated with reflux esophagitis [12].

CLINICAL PRESENTATIONS

The common signs and symptoms of GER/GERD in the pediatric population vary with age [2] and are more non-specific in younger children (Table 1 and 2). Exclusively breastfed infants regurgitate less than partially breastfed infants [6]. Symptoms of gastroesophageal reflux are most often directly related either to the consequences of emesis (e.g., poor weight gain) or a result of exposure of the esophageal epithelium to gastric contents. While an older child may present with typical symptoms (e.g., heartburn, vomiting, regurgitation) seen in adults; infants and young children [13] with GER may have non-specific symptoms of fussiness [14], irritability, crying, sleep disturbance or refusal to eat. The common symptoms of GERD such as vomiting/regurgitation, abdominal pain and cough are not predictors of presence or absence of esophagitis, however, the prevalence of feed refusal is significantly greater in erosive esophagitis versus non-erosive esophagitis [15]. GERD can be a great masquerader, as it may be suspected by dentists, ENT or pulmonary specialists if patients have atypical symptoms (e.g., dental erosion [16], nocturnal cough, stridor, wheezing, or hoarseness as the only major complaint). Usually, diagnosis of GER can be suspected by suggestive clinical history. Physical Examination is usually normal, except in Sandifer syndrome, which may be misdiagnosed as spastic torticollis.

Table 1. Signs and Symptoms of GERD in Infants and Young Children

Vomiting/ regurgitation including via naso-pharynx
Persistent crying and/or irritability/Fussiness
Poor appetite/ / Gagging/ Feeding difficulty
Back arching/ Sleep problems
Apparent life-threatening event (ALTE)
Weight loss/ Poor growth/ Failure to thrive
Recurrent pneumonia/ Wheezing/ Chronic cough/Stridor
Sore throat/ Hoarseness and/or laryngitis/ Hiccups/ Waterbrash
Sandifer syndrome (ie, posturing with opisthotonus or torticollis)
Hematemesis/Occult blood positive stools
Abdominal pain

Table 2. Signs and Symptoms in Older Children

All of the above
Retrosternal chest pain/ Heartburn
Dental erosion
Halitosis

Extra-oesophageal symptoms are thought to be common, atypical symptoms of GERD in children. A systematic review of articles in PubMed and EMBASE was conducted to investigate the prevalence of GERD in children with extra-oesophageal symptoms in children with GERD, and the effect of GERD therapies on extra-oesophageal symptoms [17]. From 18 relevant articles, the pooled weighted average prevalence of GERD in asthmatic children was 23%, compared with 4% in healthy controls from the same five studies. Health care providers should be aware that GERD is a potential trigger of asthma, although not all asthma patients with GERD experience reflux symptoms. Possible mechanisms for gastroesophageal reflux–mediated airway disease include microaspiration of gastric contents that leads to inflammation and bronchospasm, and esophageal acid–induced reflex bronchospasm . All patients with refractory asthma should be questioned about reflux symptoms, and antireflux therapy, in particular high-dose PPI therapy should be initiated if appropriate [18,19]. Referral to a gastroenterologist may be warranted.

The majority of studies evaluating the relationship between apparent life-threatening event (ALTE) and GERD did not suggest a causal relationship [2]. Seven studies reported that respiratory symptoms, sinusitis and dental erosion were significantly more prevalent in children with GERD than in controls [2]. Data from pharmacotherapeutic trials were inconclusive and provided no support for a causal relationship between GERD and extra-oesophageal symptoms. Review of pediatric guidelines suggests that possible associations exist between GERD and asthma, pneumonia, bronchiectasis, ALTE, laryngotracheitis, sinusitis and dental erosion, but causality or temporal association were not established. Moreover, the paucity of studies, small sample sizes, and varying disease definitions did not allow firm conclusions to be drawn. Most trials of GERD therapies showed no improvement in extra-oesophageal symptoms in children.

The main differential diagnoses include the surgical and anatomical abnormalities including malrotation and pyloric stenosis in patients with persistent vomiting (Table 3). Malrotation is of particular importance as it is a 'ticking time bomb' which may result in volvulous and short gut syndrome, but can be easily prevented if detected in a timely fashion. Not all cases of pyloric stenosis present with projectile vomiting, nor all cases of malrotation present with bilious vomiting. Therefore, it is always prudent to exclude a surgical condition with a radiological contrast study when suspicion is raised due to persistent emesis.

The role of Cow's milk protein intolerance (CMPI) in infantile reflux disease cannot be overemphasized, although it is predominantly evidence based. CMPI affects 3% of infants under the age of 12 months and often missed in the primary care setting [20]. Of similar significance is eosinophilic gastroenteropathy (EGE), an allergic condition mimicking GERD [21], which can be diagnosed by endoscopic histopathology of esophagus demonstrating more than 20 eosinophils per high power field. Mean age of presentation is 7 years (range 1-17) and patients often show atopy. Presenting symptoms include vomiting, retrosternal or epigastric pain, dysphagia with occasional food impaction and sleep disturbance [22].

Table 3. Differential Diagnoses of GERD in Children

Anatomic malformations: Pyloric stenosis, malrotation, antral web etc
Food Allergies/ Eosinophilic esophagitis
Peptic Ulcer Disease / Gastritis/ *Helicobacter pylori* Infection
Esophageal and/or Intestinal Motility Disorders
Irritable Bowel Syndrome
Central nervous system disorders
UTI/ Otitis media in infancy

DIAGNOSTIC EVALUATION

In most cases of gastroesophageal reflux (GER), diagnosis can be made from the history and physical examination. Conservative measures can be started empirically. However, if the presentation is atypical or if response to therapy is minimal, further evaluation is warranted. Since this review is an update of pediatric GERD, only newer and more relevant information is discussed.

Radiologic Studies

Upper GI imaging series is helpful to exclude anatomic problems of the upper GI tract including strictures, however, it is neither sensitive nor specific for GERD. Gastric scintiscan is performed using milk or formula that contains a small amount of technetium sulfur colloid, can assess gastric emptying and can reveal presence and the level of refluxate as well as for assessment of pulmonary aspiration, if it occurs during the study. Gastro-esophageal ultrasound is not a frequently used study.

pH Probe Monitoring

Intraesophageal pH probe monitoring can be accomplished by an indwelling catheter or via a wireless technique. Although a very sensitive technique, precise criteria for differentiating "physiologic" from "pathologic" gastroesophageal reflux vary in different centers [23]. Dual pH probe catheter monitoring has been used to assess both distal and proximal esophageal reflux in an attempt to correlate gastroesophageal reflux with both laryngeal and pulmonary symptoms, however, no clear consensus has emerged. The ability to establish a temporal relationship with atypical symptoms (e.g., obstructive apnea) and reflux events may be helpful [24]. Role of non-acid reflux is becoming important in evaluation many of these symptoms.

Limitations of conventional catheter-based pH testing include patient intolerance, potential for catheter migration, limitations in patients' physical and dietary activity owing to discomfort, and the relatively short term of pH studies [25]. The development of the Bravo wireless pH capsule has circumvented some of these problems and has the additional advantage of allowing 48-h recording periods, which may increase its sensitivity in the diagnosis of GERD. The Bravo pH capsule was as accurate, safe and better tolerated than the conventional pH catheter in children 4 years of age and older, when both modalities were studied simultaneously. When reflux scores during the first 24 hours were compared with the 48-hour measurements in another pediatric study, although individual variations were noted, they were not clinically significant. These observations support the use of pH-measurement for a period of 24 hours only, however, Bravo capsule allows prolonged pH monitoring under more physiologic conditions [26].

Intraluminal Esophageal Impedance

Multichannel Intraluminal esophageal Impedance is useful for detecting both acid reflux and nonacid reflux by measuring retrograde flow and its level in the esophagus [27]. It also helps to differentiate between liquid and gaseous reflux. The addition of impedance component to standard pH monitoring increases the likelihood of demonstrating an association between events and GER symptoms. It is helpful in assessing adequacy of acid suppression in patients with ongoing symptoms despite appropriate treatment. This is fast replacing routine pH monitoring.

Esophagogastroduodenoscopy (EGD) with Biopsy

This is the most useful single test to conclusively exclude other upper gastro-intestinal pathology such as Eosinophilic Esophagitis, other infectious esophagitis, *H. pylori* disease spectrum, celiac disease and other conditions. Furthermore, ability to obtain biopsies for histology examination adds to the information obtained during visualization. Inlet patch has been reported to be associated with respiratory symptoms and erosive esophagitis [28]. A recent USA cross-sectional study of individuals aged less than 18 years who underwent EGD for a primary indication of abdominal pain at two US centers between January 2002 and June 2005 showed that EGD had better diagnostic yield, in contrast with most alarm symptoms and routine laboratory tests evaluated. EGD was diagnostic in 38.1% of the 1191 of children experiencing chronic abdominal pain in this study [29].

Histologic features of reflux esophagitis include basal cell hyperplasia, extended papillae, and mucosal eosinophils. The number of mucosal eosinophils per high-powered field (hpf) is important because presence of more than 20 per hpf is suggestive of eosinophilic (allergic) esophagitis rather than peptic esophagitis [2,21,30].

TREATMENT

Since infant GER is self resolving usually, reassurance may suffice initially. Conservative measures like proper burping, upright positioning after feeding, elevating the head of the bed, and small frequent feeds can be suggested. The association of prone positioning with sudden infant death syndrome (SIDS) has made its use controversial. Obviously, the use of the prone position during infancy must be based on a careful risk-to-benefit analysis [2]. When advised, only very firm bedding material (no pillows) must be used. Bed elevation does not offer any additional advantage with the prone position, and seated positions are not recommended. Recently, left lateral decubitus position has been shown to help reflux at all ages [31], but gastric residuals in growing preterm infants were significantly less in right lateral decubitus than the prone position and left lateral decubitus [32].

Formula thickening with cereal may help when excessive vomiting is associated with suboptimal weight gain. A prethickened formula may decrease symptoms as confirmed by a recent meta-analysis [33].

Trial of a hypoallergenic formula may be considered in infants, as surprisingly, cow's milk protein intolerance is much more common underlying offender mimicking infantile GERD than it is suspected [21]. Maternal elimination of cow's milk in empiric breast-fed infants with GERD may be beneficial in some [34], however, prolonged restriction of maternal diet without objective need for such elimination may lead to impaired maternal nutrition and affect quality of life. In non-breast fed infants with persistent distress attributed to reflux esophagitis, treatment with hypoallergenic aminoacid-based formula may be an initial helpful strategy to exclude food allergies [35].

Lifestyle interventions as in adults are recommended for older children avoiding potentially refluxogenic foods , such as tomato and citrus products, fruit juices, peppermint, chocolate, and caffeine-containing beverages. Smaller portion sizes and a relatively lower fat containing diet may help. Avoidance of alcohol and tobacco should be advised when applicable. Appropriate weight management of overweight or obese children is important [2].

Frequently, life-style modifications are not enough, and in addition to conservative management, pharmacologic intervention may yield a better long-term response. A "step-up" and "step-down" approach under the care of a pediatric gastroenterologist is ideal. In "step-up" pharmacologic intervention, therapy involves progression from diet and lifestyle changes to H2 receptor antagonists (H$_2$RAs) to proton pump inhibitors (PPIs) [2]. Both classes of acid antisecretory medications have been proven safe and effective for both infants and children in reducing gastric acid output. However, its indiscriminate use and abuse is to be avoided. The majority of infants prescribed antireflux drugs, do not meet diagnostic criteria for GERD. Similarly, after improvement, every effort should be made to "step-down" the pharmacotherapy as tolerated. Careful monitoring under optimal nonsurgical therapy should be conducted before considering operative intervention.

PPIs suppress gastric acid secretion by inhibiting H+, K+ ATPase enzyme system (i.e., proton pump) at the secretory surface of the gastric parietal cell which is the final step of acid production [36-42]. The effect is dose-related and inhibits both basal and stimulated gastric acid secretion, thus increasing gastric pH. They should be administered before the first meal of the day. Children with nasogastric or gastrostomy tubes may have granules mixed in an acidic juice or suspensions for administration. The tubes must be flushed to prevent blockage. Omeprazole, lansoprazole and esomeprazole have been approved between 1-17 years of age by FDA and rabeprazole for 12-17 years old individuals based on safety and efficacy data. Efficacy and safety of pantoprazole in pediatric patients has also been reported [43].

In managing children with GERD, there is increasing evidence that they need higher dosages of acid suppressive therapy to achieve clinical response. The CYP2C19 isoform of cytochrome p450 is the principal enzyme responsible for the metabolism of PPIs; the genotypes of which are classified into three groups: extensive metabolizer, intermediate metabolizer, and poor metabolizer. The relative impact of the CYP2C19 pathway on the metabolism of PPIs has been reported to be mostly in omeprazole and esomeprazole followed by pantoprazole, lansoprazole, and the least with rabeprazole [44]. This would therefore affect the metabolic and pharmacokinetic profiles of PPIs. Recent studies have brought to light the important role that this polymorphism may play in the therapeutic effectiveness of PPIs in the treatment of GERD and its complications. Genetic polymorphisms of CYP2C19 shows marked interracial differences, with the poor metabolizer phenotype representing 2-5% of whites and up to 11-24% of adult Asian populations (Chinese 24%, Japanese 18%).

Continued long-term medical pharmacologic management of GERD with PPIs has been shown to be safe in retrospective study [45]. There have been concerns regarding effects of acid suppression leading to increased susceptibility to community acquired pneumonias [46] and possible effects on calcium homeostasis. Rebound acid hypersecretion (RAHS) has been demonstrated after 8 weeks of treatment with PPI use in adult healthy volunteers after withdrawal [47]. If RAHS induces acid-related symptoms, this might lead to PPI dependency and thus have important implications. Since this study included healthy volunteers, it prevents us from determining whether symptoms develop as a consequence of RAHS to the same degree in patients with dyspeptic symptoms. In addition, its clinical significance in *H. pylori* infected subjects is not known.

SURGICAL INTERVENTION

As pharmacotherapy has improved, the need for surgical therapy (fundoplication) has markedly decreased. However, antireflux surgery remains one of the most common surgical procedures performed during infancy and early childhood. Surgical therapy, such as laparoscopic Nissen fundoplication, is an option for patients who have failed to respond to medications, experience complications of GERD, or have elected to have surgery out of choice despite successful medication therapy. The goal of surgery is to reestablish the antireflux barrier, without creating obstruction to the food bolus. In general, the Nissen fundoplication, which is a complete 360° wrap gives better control of reflux symptoms; dysphagia and gas bloat are potential complications [2,48,49,50].

Before considering surgery, patients should be evaluated with a thorough history and physical examination, and good response to medical treatment helps to predict good outcome. The role of surgery is debated for children with atypical GERD. Maximum medical treatment including conservative and pharmacologic treatment should be done before contemplating surgical intervention and unnecessary surgeries should must be avoided.

RECENT DEVELOPMENTS

Since GERD is a heterogeneous disorder, a global evidence based consensus on the definition of GERD has been developed. Algorithms and guidelines for evaluation are available. However, management of GERD in children should be considered in the context of their age and other special circumstances, and individualized at clinician's discretion. A synopsis of guidelines for clinical practice, formulated by the joint recommendations of the North American Society for Pediatric Gastroenterlogy, Hepatology and Nutrition (NASPGHAN) and the European Society for Pediatric Gastroenterlogy, Hepatology, and Nutrition (ESPGHAN) is now available [2]. A brief summary of the recent updates of the guidelines for the management of pediatric GERD follows:

GERD in Infancy

Gastroesophageal reflux disease in infants usually presents as recurrent spitting up, crying and fussiness and excessive vomiting. In severe cases, they may fail to thrive, have feeding difficulty including choking and gagging, or respiratory complications such as acute life threatening events or apnea. Diagnostic studies for projectile vomiting include Barium contrast study or ultrasonography to exclude structural abnormalities such as malrotation and pyloric stenosis. Gastro-esophageal scintigraphy may be helpful to determine aspiration and delayed gastric emptying. Extended pH/impedance is the test of choice to evaluate acid vs. non-acid reflux disease. Similar presenting symptoms are seen with cow's milk protein intolerance (CMPI) as well.

After a suggestive history and normal physical exam, formula change and/or a trial of hypoallergenic formula is the initial step in management. Upright or left lateral position after feeding may help along with thickening of formula with cereal. Pharmacotherapy is the last resort, and includes acid suppression or prokinetic agents. The latter group of medications has not been effective. Although not approved, proton pump inhibitors have been used in infants without significant efficacy. Overall, GERD in infancy is considered to be a self resolving condition with upright posture and introduction of solids and most infants outgrow it. In a few with serious complications such as recurrent apneas, surgical fundoplication should be considered.

GERD in Older Children

Gastroesophageal reflux disease in older children mirrors the symptoms in the adult population and these symptoms usually start *de novo* in otherwise normal patients. The most common symptoms are nausea, acid taste in the mouth or regurgitation, heartburn, upper abdominal pain and sometimes with extra-esophageal symptoms. Children should be interviewed and asked some questions directly as they may not voice all their symptoms to their parents.

Diagnosis is mainly clinical. Endoscopy with biopsy should be performed in all moderate to severe cases or in patients with persistent symptoms to rule out other upper gastro-intestinal conditions such as eosinophilic esophagitis (EE) or *H. pylori* gastritis. On histology, markers of inflammation and presence of <20 eosinophils per high power field are usually more characteristic of GERD. Other available tests include pH/impedance study, bravo capsule pH monitoring. Radiologic tests are rarely needed.

Dietary and lifestyle modifications are very important. Treatment is based on decreasing the noxiousness of the refluxate by suppressing the acid using H_2 receptor antagonists (H2RAs). Efficacy of proton-pump inhibitors (PPIs) in children has been well documented, and step-up treatment to PPIs is needed frequently.

GERD in Special Populations

Children with developmental delay and cerebral palsy are at high risk for developing GERD due to multiple pre-disposing factors such as; supine posture, poor muscle tone or spasticity, esophageal dysmotility, hiatal hernia and others. Chronic lung diseases such as asthma and cystic fibrosis render children more susceptible to GERD and reflux is also more common in children with anatomical and structural abnormalities such as repaired tracheo-esophageal fistula (TEF) [2]. GERD in such children may need aggressive medical treatment. Prolonged PPI use is common and many of them need fundoplication.

Esophageal atresia (EA) is the most common congenital anomaly of the esophagus. The prevalence of esophageal symptoms and pathology were evaluated in a descriptive study of adults aged 20 years or older who had surgery for EA as infants. Individuals were assessed by using a structured questionnaire. Endoscopy was performed in 62/132 patients because of symptoms. Reflux symptoms, esophagitis, and Barrett's esophagus were common in this cohort. Close follow-up with clinical assessment and upper endoscopy for reflux symptoms or dysphagia is recommended. Transition of young adults from pediatric care to an adult gastroenterology clinic with expertise in EA appears to be highly beneficial [51].

EMERGING NATURAL HISTORY

There is an increasing awareness of the fact that GERD like other lifelong digestive diseases (i.e. Crohn's disease) may actually have its origin in childhood [52]. Pediatric GER likely shares a similar pathophysiology to adult GER, and preliminary data suggests a genetic susceptibility to GERD.

However, further studies will be necessary to confirm this hypothesis. In children, GER has a distinct presentation from that in adults, with the diagnostic work-up based upon the patient's age as well as their presenting signs and symptoms. Like their adult counterparts, the early detection and treatment of GER in children may result in better long-term outcome, improved quality-of-life, and a reduction in overall healthcare burden.

Attention has been focused on Quality of Life (QOL) issues in children and adolescents with GERD recently. The QOL in Reflux and Dyspepsia questionnaire (QOLRAD), previously validated in adults, consists of 25 questions grouped into 5 domains: emotional distress, sleep disturbance, food/drink problems, physical/social functioning, and vitality. It was administered at the baseline and after 8 weeks treatment with esomeprazole to examine the effect of GERD on health-related quality of life (HRQOL) in adolescents [41]. Baseline QOLRAD scores indicated GERD had a negative effect on the HRQOL of these adolescents, especially in the domains of vitality and emotional distress, and problems with food/drink. After esomeprazole treatment, statistically and clinically significant improvements occurred in all domains of the QOLRAD for these adolescents [53]. Self-reported Quality of life (QoL) including physical, emotional, social and school domains was assessed in children with GERD aged 5-18 and compared with both patients with other gastrointestinal conditions like constipation and inflammatory bowel disease (IBD) and healthy control children in another prospective study [54]. Self-reported QoL in children with GERD attending a tertiary paediatric gastroenterology clinic was significantly reduced compared with both healthy children and children with IBD. Such data suggest that appropriate management of these patients is needed to improve QOL in these patients. Unfortunately, there is a paucity of well-designed longitudinal studies that characterize the natural history of each of these conditions and more importantly identify individuals (i.e., children) who are at risk for serious, long-term adult sequelae.

Gastroesophageal reflux (GER), the physiological condition, and GERD, the disease, occur frequently during the first 2 yr of life. In a recent Italian study, Campanozzi et al. used Rome II criteria for infant regurgitation and demonstrated that 88% infants improved at 12 months of age and only 1 out of 210 infants remained to have GERD after 24 months of age [55]. Breast fed showed earlier resolution of symptoms [55]. Symptoms abate without treatment in 60% of infants by age 6 months, when these infants begin to assume an upright position and eat solid foods. Resolution of symptoms occurs in approximately 90% of infants by age 8-10 months. Those with persistent symptoms beyond 18 months of age may have a higher likelihood of chronic GERD [56,57].

However, commonly held "dogma" by pediatricians is the belief that the majority of these children "grew out of their GER or GERD symptoms." On the contrary, recent evidence suggests that GERD in some subjects is a chronic, potentially life-long condition that begins in childhood, and in those in whom disease onset is early, there may be a higher risk for long-term severe disease sequelae. In the first systematic, longitudinal prospective study that employed both a validated GERD symptom assessment instrument and a histological characterization of esophageal inflammation via mucosal biopsies of infants during the first year of life; objective data and symptom scores were collected at 2, 4, 6, and 12 months. At the 12-month endpoint, 10 of 19 infants completed the study without rescue medication and overall symptom scores improved in all 10 completers. However, none of the 10 completers had normalization of biopsy assessments, i.e., basal cell layer <25% and papillary height <53% of epithelial thickness. The authors concluded that although symptoms improved in more than half of infants with reflux esophagitis followed longitudinally, esophageal mucosal histology remained abnormal at the 1-yr evaluation in the absence of pharmacotherapy [58]. The lack of concordant improvement of the esophageal histology raises concern regarding sub-clinical persistence of ongoing esophageal insult, which might in the long-term, predispose the individual to GERD-related complications, such as strictures, Barrett's esophagus, and/or esophageal adenocarcinoma.

A retrospective study suggested that pediatric GER is a heterogeneous disorder and that GERD occurring after infancy may be more predictive of the presence of GERD during adulthood. The duration of gastroesophageal reflux disease (GERD) is an important factor in the development of esophageal complications. Longitudinal follow-up of a larger number of children is needed to answer the question of when classic adulthood GERD begins [59].

Whether GERD in childhood progresses or predisposes to GERD in adulthood remains unknown. The clinical course of gastroesophageal reflux disease (GERD) in children without predisposing comorbid illnesses has been evaluated. GERD in otherwise normal children can persist through adolescence and adulthood in a significant proportion of patients who continue to have GERD symptoms and signs, and use antisecretory medications [60]. Frequent GERD symptoms requiring antisecretory therapy were present in approximately half of young adults with a history of childhood GERD. The use of oral contraceptives was a risk factor for GERD symptoms in these individuals [61].

GENETICS OF PEDIATRIC GERD

Preliminary genetic studies have not established a specific locus for GERD as yet, however, physiologically and phenotypically as diverse disorder such as GERD is most likely determined by more than one locus or may have a more complicated molecular basis. Further molecular studies will enhance our understanding of its pathophysiology and management in the future.

RECENT PROGRESS

Novel GABA(B) agonist drugs have been shown by Dent et al to inhibit transient relaxations (TLESR) and currently being evaluated in clinical trials on patients with reflux disease [3]. This may be a possible breakthrough particularly for pediatric GERD patients, as safe and effective prokinetic are lacking.

CLINICAL VIGNETTES

- ♥ Gastroesophageal reflux in pediatrics is a heterogeneous disorder and is self resolving in most infants by 12 months of age. However, it older children, it tends to be more chronic.
- ♥ Anatomical abnormalities and eosinophilic esophagitis must be excluded in patients with persistent and non remitting symptoms despite treatment.
- ♥ Breast feeding and hypoallergenic formulas may be beneficial in decreasing symptoms of infantile GERD in appropriately selected patients.

- ♥ Several PPIs have been shown to be safe and efficacious in 1-17 year old children with GERD for 8-12 weeks. Retrospective studies with long term PPIs have shown them to be safe, although clinical and laboratory monitoring should be done.
- ♥ Surgical intervention should be considered judiciously after maximum medical treatment.

REFERENCES

[1] Sherman PM, Hassall E, Fagundes-Neto U, Gold BD, Kato S, Koletzko S, Orenstein S, Rudolph C, Vakil N, Vandenplas Y. A global, evidence-based consensus on the definition of gastroesophageal reflux disease in the pediatric population. *Am J Gastroenterol.* 2009 May;104(5):1278-95; quiz 1296. Epub 2009 Apr 7. Review. PubMed PMID: 19352345.

[2] Vandenplas Y, Rudolph CD, Di Lorenzo C, Hassall E, Liptak G, Mazur L, Sondheimer J, Staiano A, Thomson M, Veereman-Wauters G, Wenzl TG; Co-Chairs:; Committee Members:. Pediatric Gastroesophageal Reflux Clinical Practice Guidelines: Joint Recommendations of the North American Society of Pediatric Gastroenterology, Hepatology, and Nutrition and the European Society of Pediatric Gastroenterology, Hepatology, and Nutrition. *J Pediatr Gastroenterol Nutr.* 2009 Sep 9. [Epub ahead of print] PubMed PMID: 19745761.

[3] Dent J. Landmarks in the understanding and treatment of reflux disease. *J Gastroenterol Hepatol.* 2009 Oct; 24 Suppl3:S5-14. PMID 19799698.

[4] Orenstein SR, Peter J, Khan K, Youssef N, Hussain SZ. *Nelson Textbook of Pediatrics* (18th Edition). 2007: The Esophagus: Section 3. Hiatal hernia: Chapter 319: 1546.

[5] Pashankar DS, Corbin Z, Shah SK, Caprio S. Increased prevalence of gastroesophageal reflux symptoms in obese children evaluated in an Academic Medical Center. *JPGN. 43(5)*: 410-413, 2009.

[6] Hegar B, Dewanti NR, Kadim M, Atalas S, Firmansyah A, Vandenplas Y. Natural evolution of regurgitation in healthy infants. *Acta Paediatrica. 98(7)*: 1189-93, 2009.

[7] Deal L, Gold BD, Gremse DA, Winter HS, Peters SB, Fraga PD, Mack ME, Gaylord SM, Tolia V, Fitzgerald JF. Age-specific questionnaires distinguish GERD symptom frequency and severity in infants and young

children: development and initial validation. *J Pediatr Gastroenterol Nutr*. 2005 Aug;41(2):178-85. PubMed PMID: 6056096.

[8] Kleinman L, Revicki DA, Flood E. Validation issues in questionnaires for diagnosis and monitoring of gastroesophageal reflux disease in children. *Curr Gastroentrol Rep*. 2006 Jun; 8(3): 230-6 PMID 16764789.

[9] Malaty HM, O'Malley KJ, Abudayyeh S, Graham DY, Gilger MA. Multidimensional measure for gastroesophageal reflux disease (MM-GERD) symptoms in children: a population based study. *Acta paediatr*. 2008 Sep;97(9):1292-7 PMID 18510718.

[10] Gunasekaran TS, Dahlberg M, Ramesh P, Namachivayam G. Prevalence and associated features of gastroesophageal reflux symptoms in a Caucasian-predominant alolesceant school population. *Did Dis Sci*. 2008 Sep;53(9): 2373-9 PMID 18204971.

[11] Levine A, MiloT, Broide E, Wine E, Dala I, Boaz M, Avni Y, Shirin H. Influence of Helicobacter pylori eradication on gastroesophageal reflux symptoms and epigastric pain in children and adolescents. *Pediatrics*. 2004 Jan;113(1 Pt 1):54-8 PMID 14702447.

[12] Moon A, Solomon A, Beneck D, Cunningham-Rundles S. Positive association between Helicobacter pylori and gastroesophageal reflux disease in children. *JPGN*. 2009 Sep;49(3):283-8 PMID 19525872.

[13] Tolia V, Wuerth A, Thomas R. Gastroesophageal reflux disease: review of presenting symptoms, evaluation, management, and outcome in infants. *Dig Dis Sci*. 2003 Sep;48(9):1723-9. PubMed PMID: 14560991.

[14] Bhatia J, Parish A. GERD or not GERD: the fussy infant. *J of Perinatology*. 2009: Suppl 2:S7-11.

[15] Gupta SK, Hassall E, Chiu YL, Amer F, Heyman MB. Presenting symptoms of nonerosive and erosive esophagitis in pediatric patients. *Dig Dis Sci*. 2006 May;51(5):858-63. Epub 2006 May 23.

[16] Dahshan A, Patel H, Delaney J, Wuerth A, Thomas R, Tolia V. Gastroesophageal reflux disease and dental erosion in children. *J Pediatr*. 2002 Apr;140(4):474-8. PubMed PMID: 12006966.

[17] Tolia V, Vandenplas Y. Systematic review: the extra-oesophageal symptoms of gastro-oesophageal reflux disease in children. *Aliment Pharmacol Ther*. 2009 Feb 1;29(3):258-72. Review. PubMed PMID: 19143046.

[18]Scarupa MD, Mori N, Canning BJ. Gastroesophageal reflux disease in children with asthma: treatment implications. *Paediatr Drugs*. 2005;7:177-86.

[19] Sopo SM, Radzik D, Calvani M. Does treatment with proton pump inhibitors for gastroesophageal reflux disease (GERD) improve asthma symptoms in children with asthma and GERD? A systematic review. *J Investig Allergol Clin Immunol*. 2009;19(1):1-5.

[20]Ewing WM, Allen PJ. The diagnosis and management of cow milk protein intolerance in the primary care setting. *apaediatr Nurs*. 2005 Nov-Dec;31(6):486-93.

[21]Putnam PE, Rothenberg ME. Eosinophilic esophagitis: concepts, controversies, and evidence. *Curr Gastroenterol Rep*. 2009 Jun;11(3):220-5. Review. PubMed PMID: 19463222.

[22]Flood EM, Beusterien KM, Amonkar MM, Jurgensen CH, Dewit OE, Kahl LP, Matza LS. Patient and caregiver perspective on pediatric eosinophilic esophagitis and nelwly developed symptom questionnaires. *Curr Med Res Opin*. 2008 Dec;24(12):3369-81.

[23]Nazer D, Thomas R, Tolia V. Ethnicity and gender related differences in extended intraesophageal pH monitoring parameters in infants: a retrospective study. *BMC Pediatr*. 2005 Jul 18;5:24. PubMed PMID: 16026617; PubMed Central PMCID: PMC1188060.

[24]Tolia V, Wuerth A, Thomas R. Diagnostic interpretation of extended pH monitoring: is there a single best method? *Dig Dis Sci*. 2005 Jan;50(1):94-9. PubMed PMID: 15712644.

[25]Francavilla R, Magistà AM, Bucci N, Villirillo A, Boscarelli G, Mappa L, Leone G, Fico S, Castellaneta S, Indrio F, Lionetti E, Moramarco F, Cavallo L. Comparison of Esophageal pH and Multichannel Intraluminal Impedance Testing in Pediatric Patients With Suspected Gastroesophageal Reflux. *J Pediatr Gastroenterol Nutr*. 2009 Aug 11. [Epub ahead of print] PubMed PMID: 19680154.

[26]Croffie JM, Fitzgerald JF, Molleston JP, Gupta SK, Corkins MR, Pfefferkorn MD, Lim JR, Steiner SJ, Dadzie SK Accuracy and tolerability of the Bravo catheter-free pH capsule in patients between the ages of 4 and 18 years. *J Pediatr Gastroenterol Nutr*. 2007 Nov;45(5):559-63. PMID: 18030233.

[27] Van Wijk MP, Benninga MA, Omari TI. Role of Multichannel intraluminal impedence technique in infants and children. *JPGN. 48 (1)*: 2-12, 2009.

[28] Macha S, Reddy S, Rabah R, Thomas R, Tolia V. Inlet patch: heterotopic gastric mucosa--another contributor to supraesophageal symptoms? *J Pediatr.* 2005 Sep;147(3):379-82. PubMed PMID: 16182679.

[29] Thakkar K, Chen L, Tatevian N, Shulman RJ, McDuffie A, Tsou M, Gilger MA, El-Serag HB. Diagnostic yield of oesophagogastroduodenoscopy in children with abdominal pain. *Aliment Pharmacol Ther.* 2009 Sep 15;30(6):662-9. Epub 2009 Jul 2.PMID: 19573168.

[30] Shah A, Kagalwalla AF, Gonsalves N, Melin-Aldana H, Li BU, Hirano I. Histopathologic variability in children with eosinophilic esophagitis. *Am J Gastroenterol.* 2009 Mar;104(3):716-21. Epub 2009 Feb 10. PubMed PMID: 19209168.

[31] Martin-Du Pan RC, Benoit R, Girardier L. The role of body position and gravity in the symptoms and treatment of various medical diseases. *Swiss Med Wkly.* 2004 Sep 18;134(37-38):543-51. Review.PMID: 15551157.

[32] Cohen S, Mandel D, Mimouni FB, Solovkin L, Dollberg S. Gastric residual in growing preterm infants: effect of body position. *Am J Perinatol.* 2004 Apr;21(3):163-6.PMID: 15085500.

[33] Horvath A, Dziechciarz P, Szajewska H. The effect of thickened-feed interventions on gastroesophageal reflux in infants: systematic review and meta-analysis of randomized, controlled trials. *Pediatrics.* 2008 Dec;122(6):e1268-77. Epub 2008 Nov 10. Review. Erratum in: Pediatrics. 2009 Apr;123(4):1254. PubMed PMID: 19001038.

[34] Heine RG. Allergic gastrointestinal motility disorders in infancy and childhood. *Pediatr Allergy Immunol. 19(5)*: 383-91, 2008.

[35] Orenstein SR, McGowan JD. Efficacy of conservative therapy as taught in the primary care setting for symptoms suggesting infant gastroesophageal reflux. *J Pediatr.* 2008 Mar;152(3):310-4. Epub 2007 Nov 7. PubMed PMID: 18280832.

[36] Hassall E, Israel D, Shepherd R, Radke M, Dalväg A, Sköld B, Junghard O, Lundborg P. Omeprazole for treatment of chronic erosive esophagitis in children: a multicenter study of efficacy, safety, tolerability and dose requirements. International Pediatric Omeprazole Study Group. *J Pediatr.* 2000 Dec;137(6):800-7.PMID: 11113836.

[37] Tolia V, Ferry G, Gunasekaran T, Huang B, Keith R, Book L. Efficacy of lansoprazole in the treatment of gastroesophageal reflux disease in children. *J Pediatr Gastroenterol Nutr.* 2002;35 Suppl 4:S308-18. PubMed PMID: 12607791.

[38] Tolia V, Fitzgerald J, Hassall E, Huang B, Pilmer B, Kane R 3rd. Safety of lansoprazole in the treatment of gastroesophageal reflux disease in children. *J Pediatr Gastroenterol Nutr.* 2002;35 Suppl 4:S300-7. PubMed PMID: 12607790.

[39] Orenstein SR, Hassall E, Furmaga-Jablonska W, Atkinson S, Raanan M. Multicenter, double-blind, randomized, placebo-controlled trial assessing the efficacy and safety of proton pump inhibitor lansoprazole in infants with symptoms of gastroesophageal reflux disease. *J Pediatr.* 2009 Apr;154(4):514-520.e4. Epub 2008 Dec 3. PubMed PMID: 19054529.

[40] Gilger MA, Tolia V, Vandenplas Y, Youssef NN, Traxler B, Illueca M. Safety and tolerability of esomeprazole in children with gastroesophageal reflux disease. *J Pediatr Gastroenterol Nutr.* 2008 May;46(5):524-33. PubMed PMID: 18493207.

[41] Gold BD, Gunasekaran T, Tolia V, Wetzler G, Conter H, Traxler B, Illueca M. Safety and symptom improvement with esomeprazole in adolescents with gastroesophageal reflux disease. *J Pediatr Gastroenterol Nutr.* 2007 Nov;45(5):520-9. PubMed PMID: 18030228.

[42] Fiedorek S, Tolia V, Gold BD, Huang B, Stolle J, Lee C, Gremse D. Efficacy and safety of lansoprazole in adolescents with symptomatic erosive and non-erosive gastroesophageal reflux disease. *J Pediatr Gastroenterol Nutr.* 2005 Mar;40(3):319-27. PubMed PMID: 15735486.

[43] Tolia V, Bishop PR, Tsou VM, Gremse D, Soffer EF, Comer GM; Members of the 322 Study Group. Multicenter, randomized, double-blind study comparing 10, 20 and 40 mg pantoprazole in children (5-11 years) with symptomatic gastroesophageal reflux disease. *J Pediatr Gastroenterol Nutr.* 2006 Apr;42(4):384-91.PMID: 16641576.

[44] Horn J. Review article: relationship between the metabolism and efficacy of proton pump inhibitors--focus on rabeprazole. *Aliment Pharmacol Ther.* 2004 Nov;20 Suppl 6:11-9. PMID: 15496214.

[45] Tolia V, Boyer K. "Long-Term Proton Pump Inhibitor Use in Children: A Retrospective Review of Safety". *Dig Dis Sci.* Feb;53(2):385-93; 2008. Epub 2007 Aug 4; 2007.

[46] Canani RB, Cirillo P, Roggero P, Romano C, Malamisura B, Terrin G, Passariello A, Manguso F, Morelli L, Guarino A; Working Group on Intestinal Infections of the Italian Society of Pediatric Gastroenterology, Hepatology and Nutrition (SIGENP). Therapy with gastric acidity inhibitors increases the risk of acute gastroenteritis and community-acquired pneumonia in children. *Pediatrics*. 2006 May;117(5):e817-20. PMID: 16651285.

[47] Reimer C, Sondergaard B, Hilstod L, Bytzer P. Proton-pump inhibitor therapy induces acid-related symptoms in healthy volunteers after withdrawal of therapy. *Gastroenterology*. 2009;137:80-87. PMID: 19362552.

[48] Kane TD, Brown MF, Chen MK; Members of the APSA New Technology Committee. Position paper on laparoscopic antireflux operations in infants and children for gastroesophageal reflux disease. *J Pediatr Surg*. 2009 May;44(5):1034-40. PubMed PMID: 19433194.

[49] IPEG Standard and Safety Committee. IPEG guidelines for the surgical treatment of pediatric gastroesophageal reflux disease (GERD). *J Laparoendosc Adv Surg Tech A*. 2009 Feb;19(1):x-xiii. PubMed PMID: 19226225.

[50] Mattioli G, Bax K, Becmeur F, Esposito C, Heloury Y, Podevin G, Lima M, MacKinlay GA, Goessler A, Tovar JA, Valla J, Tuo P, Nahum L, Ottonello G, Sacco O, Gentilino V, Pini-Prato A, Caponcelli E, Jasonni V. European multicenter survey on the laparoscopic treatment of gastroesophageal reflux in patients aged less than 12 months with supraesophageal symptoms. *Surg Endosc*. 2005 Oct;19(10):1309-14. Epub 2005 Aug 11.PMID: 16151683.

[51] Deurloo JA, Ekkelkamp S, Taminiau JA, Kneepkens CM, ten Kate FW, Bartelsman JF, Legemate DA, Aronson DC. Esophagitis and Barrett esophagus after correction of esophageal atresia. *J Pediatr Surg*. 2005 Aug;40(8):1227-31.PMID: 16080923.

[52] Gold BD. Is gastroesophageal reflux disease really a life-long disease: do babies who regurgitate grow up to be adults with GERD complications? *Am J Gastroenterol*. 2006 Mar;101(3):641-4. PMID: 16542297.

[53] Gunasekaran T, Tolia V, Colletti RB, Gold BD, Traxler B, Illueca M, Crawley JA. Effects of esomeprazole treatment for gastroesophageal reflux disease on quality of life in 12- to 17-year-old adolescents: an

international health outcomes study. *BMC Gastroenterol* 2009; 9:84, MID: 19922626.

[54]Marlais M, Fishman JR, Köglmeier J, Fell JM, Rawat DJ. Reduced quality of life in children with Gastro-oesophageal reflux disease. *Acta Paediatr Nov* 2009; PMID: 19930192.

[55]Campanozzi A, Boccia G, Pensabene L, Panetta F, Marseglia A, Strisciuglio P, Barbera C, Magazzu G, Pettoello-Mantovani M, Staiano A. Prevalence and natural history of gastroesophageal reflux: pediatric prospective survey. *Pediatrics.* 2009 Mar;123(3):779-83. PMID 19255002.

[56]Martin AJ, Pratt N, Kennedy JD, Ryan P, Ruffin RE, Miles H, Marley J. Natural history and familial relationship of infant spilling to 9 years of age. *Pediatrics.* 2002 Jun; 109(6):1061-7 PMID 12042543.

[57]Nelson SP, Chen EH, Syniar GM, Christoffel KK. One-year follow-up of symptoms gastroesophageal reflux during infancy: Pediatric Practice Research Group. *Pediatrics.* 1998 Dec;102(6):E67 PMID 9832595.

[58]Orenstein SR, Shalaby TM, Kelsey SF, Frankel E. Natural history of infant reflux esophagitis: symptoms and morphometric histology during one year without pharmacotherapy. *Am J Gastroenterol.* 2006 Mar;101(3):628-40. PubMed PMID:16542296.

[59]Young RJ, Lyden E, Ward B, Vandrhoof JA, DiBaise JK. A retrospective, case-control pilot study of the natural history of pediatric gastroesophageal reflux. *Dig Dis Sci.* 2007 Feb;52(2):457-62. Pubmed PMID 17211703.

[60]El-Serag HB. Time trends of gastroesophageal reflux disease: a systematic review. *Clin Gastroenterol Hepatol.* 2007 Jan;5(1):17-26. Epub 2006 Dec 4. Review.PMID: 17142109.

[61]El-Serag HB, Richardson P, Pilgrim P, Gilger MA. Determinants of gastroesophageal reflux disease in adults with a history of childhood gastroesophageal reflux disease. *Clin Gastroenterol Hepatol.* 2007 Jun;5(6):696-701.PMID: 17544996.

In: Reflux Disease: Causes, Symptoms and …   ISBN: 978-1-61668-694-9
Editor: G. M. Esposito, pp. 97-125   © 2010 Nova Science Publishers, Inc.

Chapter IV

PARAESOPHAGEAL HERNIAS AND USE OF MESH IN LAPAROSCOPIC ANTIREFLUX PROCEDURES

Stavros A. Antoniou, Rudolph Pointner
and Frank A. Granderath
Department of General and Visceral Surgery, Center for Minimally
Invasive Surgery, Krankenhaus "Maria v. d. Aposteln",
Mönchengladbach, Germany.

ABSTRACT

Paraesophageal hernia represents a rare acquired anatomical abnormality, comprising of migration of the stomach into the thoracic cavity and folding of the latter alongside the lower esophagus in a side-by-side manner. Due to the high complication rates of this condition, operative management is essential even in the absence of reflux symptomatology. Laparoscopic techniques provide the advantage of enhanced access to the mediastinum and precise dissection of the tissue surrounding the migrated stomach. Although the first reports on the outcome of laparoscopic fundoplication for the management of paraesophageal hernias exhibited good to excellent mid- and long term results with regard to symptom remission and reflux control, high recurrence rates led to skepticism on the efficacy and durability of primary suture hiatal closure. Hernia recurrence and intrathoracic wrap migration occurs in up to 42% of patients undergoing simple hiatoplasty due to either disruption of the diaphragmatic crura muscle fibers, wrap slippage through the intact hiatus or rupture of the sutures. Intrathoracic negative and intraabdominal positive pressures represent the most determinative physiological factors for these complications. The application of prosthetic material as reinforcement of the diaphragmatic defect in cases of paraesophageal hernia resulted in a dramatic decrease of recurrence rates and has an absolute indication in this patient population. However, mesh hiatoplasty is accompanied by several foreign-body complications, including mesh erosion, dysphagia, as well as severe epigastric pain. These complications result in a significant decrease of patients' quality of life and often require surgical reintervention. Therefore, mesh hiatoplasty should be applied in selected cases, with regard to the type and the size of the hiatal hernia, the surface of the hiatal defect and individual patient characteristics. Furthermore, clinical decisions should keep up with current evidence-based trends in order to minimize complications of antireflux procedures and improve patients' quality of life.

INTRODUCTION

The introduction of laparoscopic techniques in the treatment of gastroesophageal reflux disease (GERD) during the early 1990's incurred dramatic changes in the therapeutic management of this condition. Minimally invasive trends rendered laparoscopic fundoplication an attractive alternative to medical therapy and subsequently broadened the indications for operative management of patients with chronic reflux symptomatology. However, several reports exhibited higher rates of wrap migration and hernia recurrence following laparoscopic hiatoplasty as compared to open techniques. Additionally, recurrence rates seemed to be proportionate to the size of the hiatal defect, thus making large hiatal and paraesophageal hernias one of the main and primary indications for application of prosthetic materials.

Hiatal hernias can be divided in four main types (Figures 1-3). Type I, also referred to as axial hernia, accounts for more than 95% of cases and refers to herniation of a part of the gastric cardia in the posterior mediastinum and thus the displacement of the lower esophageal sphincter above the hiatus. Negative thoracic pressure is one of the main factors contributing to reflux of gastric juice into the lower esophagus and explains the prevalence of heartburn in this patient population. Complications of this type of hernia are rare and mostly due to chronic gastroesophageal reflux. However, if the hiatal defect is large and a sufficient proportion of the gastric cardia is contained in the thoracic cavity, pressure symptomatology may result in cardiac or pulmonary complications as described below.

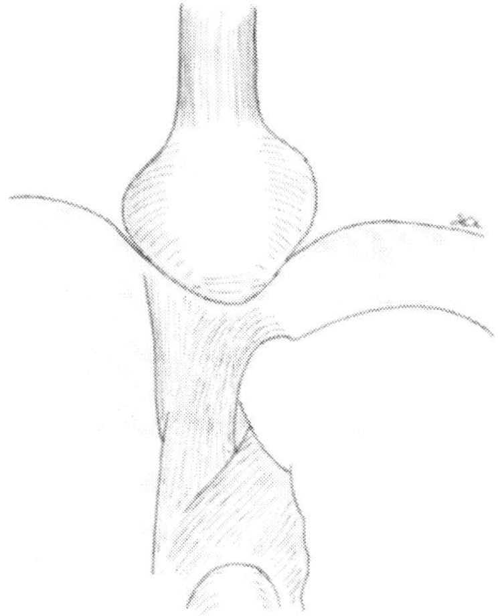

Figure 1. Type I hiatal hernia.

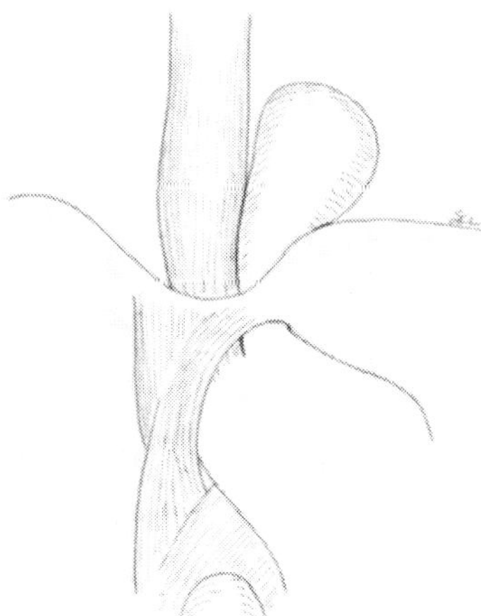

Figure 2. Type II hiatal hernia.

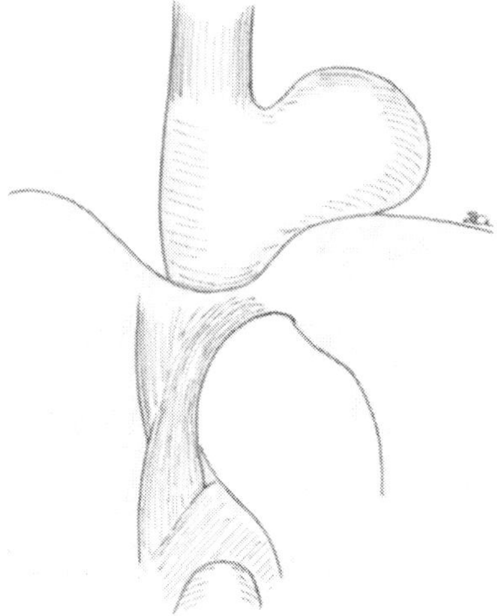

Figure 3. Type III hiatal hernia.

Type II hiatal hernia includes transposition of the gastric fundus in the mediastinum alongside the lower esophagus, leaving the gastroesophageal junction intact in its physiologic intraabdominal position. Type III hiatal hernia represents a combination of the first two types, and regards translocation of the gastric cardia in the mediastinum and folding of the gastric fundus alongside the lower esophagus. The principal risk in type II and type III hernias is strangulation of the herniated stomach, gastric volvulus and proximal stomach distention due to continuing secretion of gastric juice, with subsequent restrained blood supply, tissue necrosis and perforation. Continuous latent bleeding from gastric ulcerations represents a frequent cause of chronic anemia in this patient population and is a potentially fatal complication in case of acute excessive hemorrhage. Cardiac pressure by the translocated viscera may result in electrocardiographic changes, atrial compression, recurrent heart failure and pulmonary edema. The compromised pulmonary tissue may also result in persistent or transient dyspnoic attacks. The significance of these complications is high, considering the high prevalence of type II and type III hiatal hernias in the older population, where cardiac and pulmonary co-morbidities are prominent. In-hospital mortality of patients with untreated symptomatic paraesophageal hernias exceeds 14% and is thus an absolute indication for operative treatment [1].

Type IV hiatal hernia is the less frequently encountered type of diaphragmatic hernia. In these cases, the excessively widened hiatal defect allows herniation of more than one abdominal viscera including stomach, colon, small bowel, spleen, liver or pancreas.

PHYSIOPATHOLOGY

The pathological mechanisms contributing to relaxation of the muscular ring of the esophageal hiatus and herniation of abdominal contents into the thoracic cavity remain mostly ambiguous. Positive intraabdominal pressure and increased intragastric pressure, especially in obese patients, contribute in the mechanical stress and anatomical disruption of the esophagogastric junction and subsequently the esophageal hiatus [2]. Intrathoracic negative pressure environment may further induce traction of the stomach into the mediastinum. Fixation of the gastroesophageal junction to the preaortic fascia and the arcuate ligament is thought to prohibit cardia migration and lead to type II hiatal hernias. Rotation of the stomach around its transverse axis results in an organoaxial volvulus, also referred to as upside-down stomach. The physiological and physiopathological factors influencing the above interrelations are still elusive.

Changes in the microenvironment of the esophagus- and stomach-related ligaments and hiatal muscle fibers have not been adequately studied yet. Relaxation of the phrenoesophageal and gastrohepatic ligaments supporting the gastroesophageal junction, introduced by reduction of the proportion of the elastic fibers by more than 50% in patients with large hiatal hernias seems to be a principal factor contributing to diaphragmatic hernia pathogenesis [3]. There is also evidence that alterations in the muscle fiber system of the diaphragmatic crura play also a role in the development of hiatal hernias [4]. Further research is expected to decipher the role of tissue proteases cleaving extracellular matrix molecules, mainly type I collagen and elastin. Fragmentation of type I collagen by matrix metalloproteinases (MMP), namely MMP-1, MMP-2 and MMP-13 results in substitution of the stable type I collagen by the immature type III collagen [5]. The above interactions result in a loss of the extracellular matrix tensile strength of the transversalis fascia of inguinal hernia patients. Similar patterns have been described for abdominal aortic aneurysm pathogenesis, Marfan's syndrome and arthritic disorders. Observational studies exhibited high prevalence of inguinal hernia and kyphosis in patients with hiatal hernias, whereas neonatal and adult cases of paraesophageal hernias and Marfan's syndrome coexistence suggest a potential link between systemic connective tissue disorders and diaphragmatic herniation [6,7]. The high prevalence of paraesophageal hernias with large hiatal defects in the older population, in whom accumulated oxidative factors chronically affect extracellular matrix proteins, amplifies the theory of connective tissue degeneration as a central factor for hiatal hernia pathogenesis.

SYMPTOMS AND SIGNS

Hiatal hernia symptomatology often varies according to the type of the anatomic abnormality. Type I hernia can be either asymptomatic or accompanied by typical reflux symptomatology, mainly heartburn and regurgitation; however, epigastric pain, asthma-like symptomatology and dysphagia may be also encountered in these patients.

Paraesophageal hernias are characterized by a wider spectrum of symptoms with a higher prevalence of chest and epigastric pain. The latter is either constant or arises suddenly postprandial and can be accompanied by nausea and/or vomiting. Dysphagia is attributed to the constrained esophageal or gastric lumen at the hiatus level due to the herniated gastric tissue. Anemia is present in one third of patients with type II hernias secondary to gastric mucosa ulceration at hiatus pressure sites. Loss of weight can be either a result of inappetence due to recurrent postprandial dyspeptic symptomatology or a manifestation of chronic anemia. Clinical examination does not provide valuable information, besides the existence of bowel sounds or the decrease of breath sounds peristernal and elimination of the Traube's space.

Acute symptoms are mostly associated to severe complications of paraesophageal hernias. Patients with gastric strangulation often present with acute or subacute retrosternal or/and epigastric pain and severe dysphagia; vomiting and aspiration is a frequent sign in these patients. Gastric hemorrhage may present as hematemesis or melena, whereas in extremely rare cases bleeding will result in a fall of the hematocrit and oligaemic shock. Signs of mediastinitis or peritonitis may be present when gastric perforation occurs.

DIAGNOSTIC WORKUP

Diagnostic tools include chest X-ray, upper gastrointestinal tract contrast series, endoscopy and computed tomography. Chest X-ray usually provides the diagnosis in large hernias, as the gastric bubble is located within the thoracic cavity behind the cardiac silhouette. Free mediastinal air indicates gastric perforation and is a surgical emergency. Barium esophagogastric studies represent the main diagnostic tool, with the typical clepsydra sign and the air-fluid intrathoracic level being pathognomonic. Barium swallow provides also information regarding the type and the size of the hernia and the degree of gastroesophageal reflux. In esophagogastroscopy, the gastric cardia will be detected superior to the stenotic area provided by the diaphragmatic crura; inversion of the endoscope at this level reveals the opening of the paraesophageal hernia. Typical esophagitis or Barrett's mucosa signs may be also present.

The above diagnostic tools are essential in order to preoperatively evaluate the extent of the anatomical abnormality and exclude premalignant and malignant lesions. Manometry and pH-studies are useful for the preoperative assessment of the esophageal motility and the presence of reflux, but may be technically unfeasible in large paraesophageal hernias. Additionally, chest and upper abdomen computed tomography (CT) may be obtained in complex cases. Furthermore, CT is mandatory in the presence of acute symptomatology, provided that the patient is hemodynamically stable. Gastric wall edema indicates acute ischemia and free mediastinal air suggests gastric perforation. Electrocardiogram and cardiac enzymes may be essential in the initial assessment of patients with acute symptomatology and aid in the differential diagnosis of cardiac pathology.

SURGICAL TREATMENT

It is generally agreed that surgery is a safe and effective option for patients with mild symptomatology substantially influencing their quality of life. Operative treatment is also indicated in the presence of severe reflux, dysphagia or aspiration-induced symptomatology. Furthermore, cardiac and pneumonic pressure symptoms are not subject to conservative measures due to the associated potentially life-threatening complications. Asymptomatic individuals and patients with mild symptomatology not affecting their quality of life may be either treated operatively or followed conservatively. Although emergency surgery has a higher mortality rate in comparison to elective hernia repair (5.4% vs. 1.38% respectively), a pooled analysis of 21 studies demonstrated similar risks for surgical death due to paraesophageal hernia repair either treated electively or by watchful waiting and surgery when acute symptoms occur [8]. The results of the above analysis also suggest that elective surgery is more beneficial for younger patients as compared to older individuals. However, emergency procedures for strangulated hernias may require an open approach and occasionally organ resection, which can contribute to a significant morbidity in the older population. Thus, concomitant morbidity, quality-adjusted life expectancy and the surgeon's clinical discretion will allow optimal decisions with regard to the choice for surgical intervention.

Minimally invasive techniques have become the standard of care in the treatment of hiatal hernias during the past two decades. Unless a contraindication for the application of pneumoperitoneum exists, elective hiatal hernias shall be approached laparoscopically, provided that the surgeon has exceeded the learning curve. It is generally accepted that laparoscopic techniques allow higher dissection and improved visibility of the lower mediastinum. Furthermore, laparoscopic treatment of paraesophageal hernias results in a lower morbidity and shorter hospital stay as compared to open repair [9]. The above facts are of great importance, considering that the majority of large paraesophageal hernias are encountered in the older population with often significant coexisting morbidities. However, recurrence rates are unacceptably high and can reach up to 42% when primary suture hiatoplasty is performed [10]. Therefore mesh application is generally considered an indication for type II and type III hernias.

Technical Details

Paraesophageal hernia repair follows the basic principles of laparoscopic antireflux procedures; special care must be given to salient modifications which are essential for optimal operative conditions and safe tissue dissection. The working trocars are placed in the typical positions, whereas the camera port may be placed more cephalad on the midline in order to optically access the mediastinal space. Alternatively, the camera port may be inserted through the left rectus muscle in order to avoid the falciform ligament. Adequate reverse Trendelenburg position will allow better exposition of the upper abdomen and hiatus.

Hernia Reduction and Crural Dissection

The herniated stomach is reduced applying smooth traction using the atraumatic graspers. Initial dissection begins with the division of the gastrohepatic ligament using the ultrasonic shears. When the right crus is reached, blunt dissection of the avascular connective tissue between the right crus and the esophagus provides a safe plan of the right lower mediastinal area. Similarly, dissection continues between the esophagus and the crural arch and then on the left side, between the esophagus and the left crus. Dissection on this side may be challenged by the presence of the short gastric vessels, extending from the intrathoracic greater curvature to the spleen. Care must be given to gentle manipulation of the diaphragmatic crura; maintenance of their peritoneal coat preserves an additional substrate for the hiatorrhaphy. As parts of the gastric wall are being freed, returning to previous steps (i.e. right-side and pre-esophageal dissection) will allow a homogenous circular preparation. Moreover, continued gastric traction with an atraumatic grasper provides simultaneous traction of the hernia sac into the peritoneal cavity. Further mediastinal dissection eventually guides to the lower esophagus; the main risk at this point is esophagus laceration. The hernia sac should be excised if visibility and safe dissection is compromised. Limited hemorrhage can be expected with extended mediastinal dissection and is usually controlled by temporary pressure application.

When adequate pre-esophageal plan is achieved, the dissection continues dorsal to the esophagus from the right side until the left crus is reached. Tight attachments of the upper pole of the spleen to the left crus can render gastric dissection difficult and hazardous. Cautery application of these peritoneal reflections ought to be performed with right lateral traction of the stomach; division of the short gastric vessels may be at this point essential. Further dissection of the periesophageal attachments in the mediastinum may be necessary until 2-4cm of the lower esophagus are obtained without tension in the peritoneal cavity. Bougie dilator must be avoided, as perforation has been reported to occur in up to 4% of patients.

Crural Repair

After complete hernia reduction, the diaphragmatic crura are approached with the application of 2-4 interrupted non-absorbable sutures. Pledget reinforcement may be essential if the crural tissue is excessively thin. Crural approximation must begin dorsally and proceed ventrally; this ensures minimal tension and disruption of the crural muscle fibers. As recurrences often occur due to muscle fiber disruption, the "bites" of the stitches should include at least 1.5cm of each crus, considering the magnifying attribute of the laparoscope. Some surgeons omit the latter step and proceed straight with "tension-free" mesh application. Mesh fixation is performed using clips, tacks, or sutures. Howsoever, fixation material ought to be placed with extreme caution regarding the underlying pericardium; although rare, the associated complications can be fatal.

Stomach Management

There is no consensus regarding the management of the reduced stomach. Extensive dissection of the periesophageal and perigastric tissue challenges the natural antireflux barrier. Fundoplication serves both for preventing hernia recurrence and reestablishing the gastroesophageal functional barrier. Gastropexy stabilizes the body of the stomach to the abdominal wall or the diaphragm and can prevent recurrence and axial rotation. Gastrostomy may be an expedient option for older patients with poor nutritional status. If adequate esophageal length cannot be obtained after extensive mediastinal dissection, Collis gastroplasty with the use of a linear stapler introduced abdominally or transthoracically is the last operative option. Technical success of the procedure depends highly on sufficient gastric mobilization and correct thoracic trocar placement through the third or fourth right intercostal space. This procedure will be necessary in less than 3% of hiatal hernia patients, as adequate mediastinal dissection will provide 2-3cm esophageal length in the vast majority of cases. Furthermore, it should be highlighted that the procedure is technically difficult and demanding even for experienced laparoscopic surgeons, and carries lower reflux control rates as compared to laparoscopic fundoplication [11].

Complications

Complications of laparoscopic paraesophageal hernia repair with mesh reinforcement occur due to intraoperative injury, foreign body reaction and fibrosis, or disruption of the fundoplication or the hiatoplasty. A review of 19 studies enrolling a cumulative number of 1380 patients exhibited an overall morbidity rate of 5% and a mortality rate of 1% [12].

Traumatic visceral injuries may reach up to 11% of laparoscopic paraesophageal hernia repairs [13]. Iatrogenic gastric serosa injuries and perforations can be usually managed laparoscopically, whereas esophageal lacerations caused by bougie insertion or tissue dissection is usually subject to open conversion, since a subsequent mediastinitis carries high mortality rates. Vagal nerve injuries are rarely recognized intraoperatively and may present with prolonged gastric atony and gastric dilatation during the first two postoperative days. Mesh fixation on the left hemidiaphragm rarely results in traumatic pericardial, myocardial or coronary injury with subsequent cardiac tamponade, arrhythmia or/and acute cardiac ischemia [14]; therefore, fixation tacks should be used sparely and cautious with respect to the underlying structures. It is advised to apply an ideal pressure depending on the position on the diaphragm, the type of the prosthetic material, tissue resistance and heart pulsation. The diaphragmatic area more susceptible to full-thickness penetration and pericardial injury during mesh fixation is depicted on Figure 4.

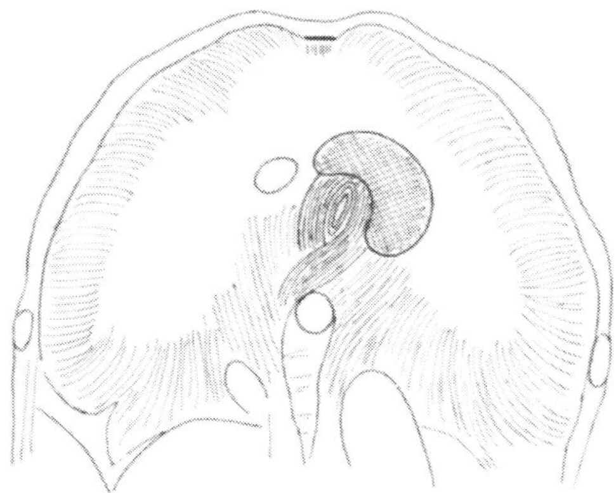

Figure 4. Diaphragmatic area most susceptible to penetration and cardiac injury during mesh fixation.

Symptoms of persistent dysphagia, heartburn, and chest and epigastric pain should alert for potential late postoperative complications [15]. Prosthetic material erosion or migration into the esophageal lumen has an incidence of 0-0.49% in large series [16,17]. No risk factors have been identified to date, while polypropylene meshes are considered to be the most irritative to the exposed esophageal tissue. The evaluation of evolutionary prosthetic materials, as collagen-coated polyester and porcine-derived biological meshes is difficult due to the low incidence of these complications. Patients will present with persistent or new onset dysphagia, regurgitation and/or epigastric pain usually within the first postoperative year. As it has been shown that early postoperative dysphagia tends to gradually relinquish [18], laparoscopic re-fundoplication should be performed as late as possible. The diagnosis of mesh erosion is made by esophagoscopy, while barium esophagographic studies may also reveal a linear stenotic area in the lower esophagus. In some patients the origin of the persisting symptomatology will be established only by laparoscopy. Persistent or new-presenting dysphagia can also occur due to visceral erosion by Teflon pledgets; this is also an infrequently encountered complication, with an incidence of 0.09% in a series of 1175 patients [19]. The same symptomatology may also occur due to mesh-induced fibrosis around the lower esophagus. These fibrotic processes may appear as 1-3cm in length stenotic areas along the lower esophagus, the condition is however difficult to be distinguished from mesh erosion. Esophagoscopy and/or exploratory laparoscopy are indicated in these cases and will provide the differential diagnosis in most cases.

Hiatal hernia recurrence either as fundic wrap migration or as disruption of the fundoplication accounts for the majority of anatomic complications requiring revisional surgery [20]. Recurrence rates following laparoscopic paraesophageal hernia repair with simple suture hiatoplasty may reach up to 42% [10]. The majority of cases are however asymptomatic and are encountered in postoperative routine studies. Operation-independent factors for anatomical failure of both simple suture and mesh reinforced hiatoplasty include vomiting and heavy lifting during the early postoperative period; however, rapid return to everyday activities has not been proved to be a risk factor for early recurrence. Operative factors for failure seem to depend on the applied technique of crural repair (Table 1). Disruption of the crural muscle fibers can be obviated by preserving the peritoneal sheet during dissection and by applying "big bites" on each crus, considering that the magnification effect of the laparoscope may overestimate tissue inclusion in the hiatorrhaphy. Suture disruption can be prevented by the use of >2/0 nonabsorbable sutures and secure knotting. Herniation through a non-disrupted cruroplasty is perhaps the most frequent cause of paraesophageal hernia recurrence. Sac excision seems to be associated with lower recurrence rates, since it allows extended esophageal mobilization [21]. If hernia recurrence occurs through a previous primary suture hiatoplasty, the use of prosthetic material would probably prevent this complication. Large hernias with a hiatal defect >6cm are subject to mesh hiatoplasty; furthermore, several authors recommend mesh application for hiatal defects >5cm or even the routine use of prosthetic materials in laparoscopic antireflux procedures. A more modest approach proposes the calculation of the hiatal defect and the tailored hiatoplasty according to the size of the interhiatal area. Indeed, large hiatal defects may be present in axial as well as in paraesophageal hernias, therefore, the exclusion of patients with type I hernia and coexisting large hiatal defects from prosthetic reinforcement techniques does not seem reasonable. The protocol of Table 2 provided a recurrence rate of 1.8% in a mean follow-up period of 6.3 months [22].

Table 1. Operative factors for failure following laparoscopic hiatoplasty

Reasons for failure	How to avoid
• Crural disrupture	• Preservation of the peritoneal sheet
	• Application of big suture ' bites"
• Suture disruption	• Use of non-absorbable sutures > 2/0
• Herniation through an intact repair	• Adequate esophageal mobilization
	• Sac excision
	• Mesh application

Revisional Fundoplication

Reoperation following failed paraesophageal hernia repair is applied either for recurrent or for new-presenting symptoms of dysphagia, regurgitation and/or heartburn, or anatomical failure of the fundoplication or the hiatoplasty.

Table 2. Proposed protocol of hiatal hernia repair

Hiatal surface area	Hiatal closure
<4cm^2	Simple sutures
>4cm^2	Simple sutures 1x3 onlay mesh
>8cm^2	Tension-free hiatoplasty

Although the current literature provides sufficient data on the outcome of revisional surgery for recurrent or new onset symptomatology with satisfactory long-term results [23,24], limited evidence exists with regard to the efficacy and durability of reoperation for fundic wrap migration or hernia recurrence. In a series of 33 patients with hiatal hernia recurrence undergoing laparoscopic re-fundoplication, satisfactory long-term results with a significant improvement of patients' quality of life and a recurrence rate as low as 6% were achieved [25].

Additionally, revisional surgery with mesh reinforcement seems a safe and effective option for patients with a previous failed simple suture hiatoplasty for reflux symptomatology. In a prospective study of 24 symptomatic patients with wrap migration, laparoscopic fundoplication with circular mesh hiatoplasty provided a significant improvement of postoperative functional studies with no recurrence in a follow-up period of 12 months [26]. Although further studies are necessary to further evaluate the postoperative symptomatic outcome in these patients, current data support the routine mesh reinforcement for patients with hernia recurrence following laparoscopic fundoplication for paraesophageal hernias or GERD.

Revisional surgery for mesh erosion or migration into the esophageal lumen is often difficult due to inflammatory tissue reaction and chronic fibrosis surrounding the repaired hiatus. Frequently encountered findings on reoperation are dense periesophageal fibrosis and mesh adherence on the diaphragmatic crura and the esophageal wall. The above render tissue dissection and mesh excision hazardous; the threshold for open conversion should thus be low. Data on operative complications are insufficient due to the rarity of foreign material complications.

CONTROVERSIAL ISSUES

Removal of the Hernia Sac

The hernia sac consists of the peritoneal sheet of the gastroesophageal junction; chronic distention of the latter due to diaphragmatic herniation results in an umbrella- or coat-like formation. Esophageal access and mobilization may be significantly challenged by the hernia sac which lies distended in the thoracic cavity while pneumoperitoneum is applied. Surgical experience suggests that excision of the sac usually provides optimal conditions for visualization of the mediastinum, adequate esophageal mobilization and sufficient retraction into the peritoneal cavity, thus avoiding an unnecessary Collis gastroplasty. For these reasons routine excision of the hernia sac is proposed by most authors, although data evaluating the operative outcome and morbidity are not available to date.

Type and Shape of the Mesh

The ideal mesh is easy to handle, creates a steady and durable complex with the diaphragmatic crura, provides durability, is resistant to infection and long-term contraction and lacks erosive effects on intraabdominal viscera. Polypropylene mesh (Prolene, Ethicon; Surgipro, Covidien) is used by many surgeons for its attribute of firmly attaching to the underlying crura, resulting in a steady complex. However, this material has an erosive effect on exposed esophageal and gastric tissue and several cases of polypropylene erosion or migration into the esophagus have been reported. Furthermore, the use of a small 1x3cm polypropylene mesh in a prospective cohort of 170 patients with reflux symptomatology and/or paraesophageal hernia resulted in a clinically manifested wrap herniation in only 0.7% of patients and no foreign body complications over a follow-up period of 12 months [29] Another prospective study of 67 patients with reflux symptomatology exhibited no hernia recurrence or complications related to polypropylene mesh application in a mean follow-up period of 22 months [27]. A retrospective review of 44 individuals with paraesophageal hernia and polypropylene mesh hiatoplasty provided similar results [30].

Polytetrafluoroethylene (PTFE) is considered to induce less adhesive reactions than polypropylene, but exhibits an increased possibility of tissue erosion, while ePTFE (Goretex, Gore) and polypropylene/ePTFE meshes (Composix, Bard) provide the advantage of encapsulation and neo-mesothelialization [31], thus becoming self-isolated from the exposed esophageal and gastric tissue. Polyester collagen-coated mesh (Parietex, Covidien) was designed to provide tissue in-growth on the polyester side and protect the contacting viscera on the other side. Nevertheless, esophageal fibrosis and ischemia, gastric and esophageal erosion have been also described for this material. The evolution of several other combinations of synthetic and absorbable materials indicates the difficulty in eliminating mesh-induced tissue reactions. Promising perspectives are provided by a porcine-derived small intestine submucosa prosthetic material (Surgisis, Cook), however without an established durability and long-term results to date [32]. Raw retrospective data exhibit a trend towards esophageal stenosis for biologic materials in contrast to mesh erosion for polypropylene and PTFE meshes [15]. Recent studies have also evaluated a novel titanium-coated polypropylene mesh (TiMesh, Medizintechnik) in hiatal hernia repair.

Different mesh shapes were also designed aiming at minimizing complications and increasing the durability of the hiatoplasty. However, the increasing variety of mesh shapes is difficult to be evaluated, due to the existence of several factors influencing clinical results, as the type of the prosthetic material, the surgical technique, and the wide range of hiatal defects included in the studies. Prosthetic meshes are distinguished in preesophageal, retroesophageal and circular. The latter have been developed due to the observation that hiatal hernia recurrence may occur posterior as well as anterior to the esophagus. It remains however elusive whether they provide lower recurrence rates with similar complication and dysphagia rates. Figures 5a-i depict the most frequently applied techniques of hiatoplasty with the corresponding mesh shapes.

Simple Reinforcement or Tension-free Hiatoplasty

The fundamental mechanism of hiatal hernia recurrence is disruption of the muscular tissue suture sites due to acute excessive or chronic tension on

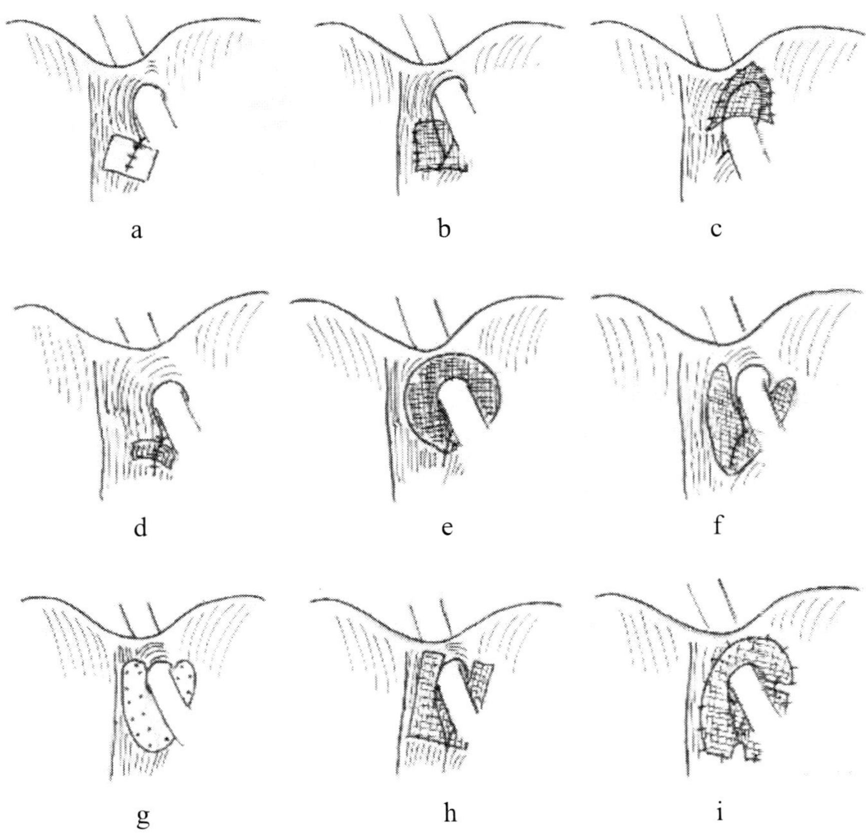

Figures 5a-i. Techniques of hiatoplasty with several mesh types. a. posterior onlay; b. posterior "tension-free"; c. anterior "tension-free"; d. posterior onlay with a 1x3cm polypropylene mesh; e. posterior hiatoplasty with circular polypropylene mesh; f. posterior "tension-free" with a V-shaped PTFE/ePTFE mesh (Crurasoft); g. posterior onlay with a V-shaped polyester collagen-coated mesh (Parietex); h. posterior "tension-free" with a U-shaped small intestine submucosa mesh (Surgisis); i. "tension-free" with an A-shaped polypropylene mesh.

the hiatoplasty by positive intraabdominal pressures. In order to diminish this tension and prevent hiatal disruption, "tension-free" hiatoplasty techniques with "bridge application" of prosthetic material without primary hiatorraphy were proposed. Anterior and posterior "tension-free" techniques were described in a few clinical studies and provided satisfactory results with regard to hernia recurrence [27]. A technique of mesh hiatus reinforcement with a relaxing incision on the diaphragm in cases where "tension-free" hiatoplasty cannot be achieved has also been also proposed [28]. Studies supporting the above techniques are however lacking long-term follow-up and high level of evidence. The tension applied on the diaphragmatic crura during every-day activities has not been measured to date and it is unknown how much of this tension is spared by the above techniques. A schematic model is depicted on Figure 6, showing that a theoretic advantage of less tension by the onlay technique may be counterbalanced by a larger mesh-free area. Current clinical data are too limited to support or discommend this theory. Onlay mesh hiatal repair, i.e. primary crurorrhaphy with subsequent prosthetic material application, remains the most popular technique of hiatal repair with well-established long-term results.

Application of an Antireflux Procedure

Mesh hiatoplasty is routinely followed by the management of the reduced stomach by means of either fundoplication or fundic anchorage to the diaphragm or the anterior abdominal wall. There are currently no clear guidelines with regard to stomach management, whereas some investigators suggest the application of fundoplication only in patients with pathologic preoperative pH-studies, suggesting that the creation of a fundic wrap contributes to postoperative dysphagia. However, there is evidence that the wrap itself does not have a significant effect on postoperative dysphagia, as does the hiatal closure [33]. Furthermore, the reliability of pH-studies in cases of large paraesophageal hernias is questionable, and the changes regarding the physiological and anatomical antireflux mechanisms in the abdominal environment after hernia reduction and extensive periesophageal dissection have not been adequately studied yet, they seem however to be partly impaired. Indeed, reflux symptomatology rates may reach up to 60% when fundoplication is omitted after paraesophageal hernia reduction and mesh hiatoplasty. Gastropexy is also thought to have an antireflux effect, whereas it can prevent hernia recurrence and organoaxial rotation. In a study of 354 laparoscopic paraesophageal hernia repairs, complication rates for gastropexy and fundoplication were 9.7% and 17.1%, respectively. Furthermore, in patients aged >70 years, gastropexy had a morbidity rate of 38.8% compared to 11.9% for fundoplication [34].

Routine use of Mesh in Antireflux Procedures

Higher recurrence rates complicating laparoscopic fundoplication as compared to open repair, prompted several investigators to examine the safety and efficacy of routine prosthetic material application for esophageal hiatus reinforcement. In a large prospective study of 531 gastroesophageal reflux patients, recurrence rates were significantly lower for mesh hiatoplasty than simple suture hiatal closure in a follow-up period of 12 months [29]. Although dysphagia was encountered more frequently in mesh-treated patients during the early postoperative period, this symptom tended to resolve within the first postoperative year and was similar for the two groups at 1-year follow-up. Similarly, a prospective randomized trial of mesh application or simple suture hiatoplsty in patients with reflux disease exhibited a significantly lower recurrence rate for the mesh group [35].

On the other hand, mesh related complications led to skepticism regarding routine application of prosthetic material in reflux disease patients. Although it seems that most of these complications, and especially foreign material reactions, occur during the first two postoperative years, long-term efficacy and safety have not been evaluated yet. Furthermore, revisional operations in patients with wrap herniation or hernia recurrence may require extensive and difficult dissection in a fibrotic environment, or even esophageal and gastric resection. In the lack of substantial long-term and subjective evidence, the tailored approach according to the size of the hiatal defect seems reasonable. The outcome of studies evaluating mesh-reinforced hiatal closure is shown in Table 3.

Future Perspectives

Evidence regarding paraesophageal hernia treatment and prosthetic mesh reinforcement is mostly scarce and based on small patient series. Multicenter prospective cohort studies are expected to decipher the issues addressed below.

Table 3. Results of laparoscopic hiatal repair with mesh hiatoplasty

Author	Year of publication	Type of study	Indications	Material used	Technique	No. of patients	Follow-up	Complications*	Recurrence	Dysphagia †
Willekes et al. [36]	1997	NR	Paraesophageal hernia, defects >2cm from the esophagus to the hiatal edge	ePTFE	posterior onlay, U-shaped	30	NR	13%	0%	3.3%
Carlson et al. [37]	1999	RCT	Hiatal defect >8cm	PTFE	posterior onlay	15	12-36mo	6.7%	0%	NR
Basso et al. [27]	2000	Prosp	GERD, hiatal hernia	Polypropylene	posterior "tension-free", 3x4cm mesh	67	mean, 22.5mo	0%	0%	NR
Frantzides et al. [38]	2002	RCT	Hiatal defect >8cm	PTFE	posterior hiatorrhaphy, circular mesh	36	mean, 3.3y	0%	0%	NR
Kamolz et al. [18]	2002	Prosp	GERD	Polypropylene	posterior onlay, 1x3cm mesh	100	1y	1%	1%	4.8%
Granderath et al. [39]	2002	Prosp	GERD	Polypropylene	posterior onlay, 1x3cm mesh	170	mean, 16 mo	NR	0.6%	4.4%
Champion and Rock [40]	2003	Retro	Hiatal defect >5cm	Polypropylene	posterior onlay, 3x5cm mesh	52	mean, 25 mo	0%	1.9%	3.8%
Granderath et al. [26]	2003	Prosp	Hernia recurrence	Polypropylene	posterior hiatorrhaphy, 10x15cm circular mesh	24	1 y	NR	0%	NR

Granderath et al. [35]	2005	RCT	GERD, hiatal hernia	Polypropylene	posterior onlay, 1x3cm mesh	100	1y	NR	8%	4%
Gryska et al. [41]	2005	Retro	GERD, hiatal hernia, hernia recurrence	PTFE or PTFE/ePTFE	posterior "tension-free", V-shaped	135	mean, 64 mo	8%	0.7%	1.5%
Granderath et al. [42]	2006	RCT	GERD	Polypropylene	posterior onlay, 1x3cm mesh	20	1y	NR	NR	5%
Kepenekci [43]	2007	Prosp	GERD	Polypropylene	posterior onlay, 1x2x3cm	176	mean, 60 mo	NR	1.8%	NR
Zanninotto et al. [44]	2007	Retro	Large type III hernia	Polypropylene and ePTFE	posterior hiatorrhaphy, 7.5cm circular mesh	35	median, 33 mo	NR	8.6%	NR
Lubezky et al. [45]	2007	Retro	Large paraesophageal hernia	PTFE or ePTFE or polyester	posterior and anterior hiatorrhaphy, circular mesh	44	mean, 28.4 mo	10.2%	35.6%	13%
			Recurrent paraesophageal hernia			15				
Jacobs et al. [46]	2007	Retro	NR	porcine-derived small intestine submucosa	posterior onlay	127	Median, 3.2y	1.6%		
Lee et al. [47]	2007	Retro	Hiatal and recurrent hernias	Human acellular dermal matrix	posterior onlay	17	mean, 14.4 mo	5.9%	12%	6%

Table 3. (Continued)

Granderath et al. [22]	2007	Prosp	Hiatal surface area >4cm^2	Polypropylene	posterior onlay, 1x3cm mesh	12	mean, 6.3 mo	NR	0%	0%
			Hiatal surface area >4cm^2	Polyester collagen-coated	Posterior, V-shaped	5				
			Hiatal surface area >8cm^2	PTFE/ePTFE	posterior "tension-free"	6				
Hazebroek et al. [48]	2008	Prosp	Large hiatal hernia	Titanium-coated polypropylene mesh (TiMesh)	posterior onlay, 4x6cm mesh	18	2 y	11.1%	0%	0%
Granderath et al. [25]	2008	Prosp	Symptom recurrence after laparoscopic antireflux surgery	Polypropylene	posterior hiatorrhaphy, 10x15cm circular mesh	33	5 y	NR	6%	6%
Lee et al. [49]	2008	Retro	Large hiatal hernia	Human acellular dermal matrix	posterior onlay, 4x7 mesh	52	median, 16	7.7%	3.8%	NR
Varga et al. [50]	2008	Prosp	Large paraesophageal hernia	Teres ligament	posterior onlay	26	1 y	11.5%	15.3%	NR
Zehetner et al. [51]	2009	Retro	Intrathoracic stomach	Vicryl	posterior onlay, application of BioGlue	30	1 y	8.6%	6.7%	NR

Soricelli et al. [17]	2009	Retro	GERD	Polypropylene	posterior "tension-free", 3x4cm mesh	113	mean, 89 mo	1.8%	2.4%	NR
				Polypropylene	posterior onlay	91		3.3%	1.8%	NR
Müller-Stich et al. [52]	2009	Retro	GERD	Polypropylene	posterior hiatorrhaphy, circular mesh, anterior cardiopexy	306	mean, 52	6%	5%	2%
Hazelbroek et al. [53]	2009	Prosp	Large hiatal hernia	ePTFE	posterior onlay of mesh pledgets	17	2 y	23.5%	0%	0%

*major complications
† new arising dysphagia

The management of asymptomatic individuals and patients with symptomatology with no influence on their quality of life is not well defined. Although current data tend to support the operative management, the identification of patient subgroups with low risks for severe complications of paraesophageal hernias will provide a more sophisticated approach of the condition. Furthermore, patient-specific indications for prosthetic material application will decrease foreign-body-related complications and improve short-term dysphagia rates. The evolution of novel prosthetic materials as well as the long-term evaluation of durability and complications of currently used meshes is expected to redefine the guidelines for hiatal closure. The application of "tension-free" or simple reinforced hiatoplasty and the definition of case-specific indications for gastropexy or fundoplication are yet to be evaluated.

CONCLUSION

The introduction of minimally invasive techniques in general surgery incurred a dramatic increase in the number of laparoscopic fundoplications and broadened the indications for operative management of GERD and hiatal hernias. High recurrence rates of laparoscopic primary hiatoplasty led to the evolution of prosthetic materials for reinforcement of the esophageal hiatus. The application of mesh-reinforced hiatal closure led to a significant improvement of short- and mid-term results, but also underscored the eventuality of foreign-material related complications and higher early postoperative dysphagia rates. In a constantly evolving research field, prospective cohort studies are expected to identify those patients who are more likely to benefit from mesh hiatoplasty. Additionally, the evolution of novel prosthetic materials is expected to minimize mesh-related complications and improve postoperative dysphagia rates.

REFERENCES

[1] Sihvo, E.I.; Salo, J.A.; Räsänen, J.V.; Rantanen T.K. (2009). Fatal complications of adult paraesophageal hernia: A population-based study. *J Thorac Cardiovasc Surg, 137,* 419-24.

[2]   Friedenberg F.K., Xanthopoulos M., Foster G.D., Richter J.E. (2008). The association between gastroesophageal reflux disease and obesity. *Am J Gastroenterol, 103*, 2111-22.

[3]   Curci J.A., Melman L.M., Thompson R.W., Soper N.J., Matthews B.D. (2008). Elastic fiber depletion in the supporting ligaments of the gastroesophageal junction: a structural basis for the development of hiatal hernia. *J Am Coll Surg, 207*, 191-196.

[4]   Fei L., del Genio G., Rossetti G., Sampaolo S., Moccia F., Trapani V., Cimmino M., del Genio A (2008). Hiatal hernia recurrence: surgical complication or disease? Electron microscope findings of the diaphragmatic pillars. *J Gastrointest Surg, 13*, 459-64.

[5]   Antoniou S.A., Antoniou G.A., Granderath F.A., Simopoulos C. (2009) The role of matrix metalloproteinases in the pathogenesis of abdominal wall hernias. *Eur J Clin Invest, 39*, 953-9.

[6]   Ruhl C.E., Everhart J.E. (2007) Risk factors for inguinal hernia among adults in the US population. *Am J Epidemiol, 165*, 1154-61.

[7]   Polomsky M., Siddall K.A., Salvador R., Dubecz A., Donahue L.A., Raymond D., Jones C., Watson T.J., Peters J.H. (2009) Association of kyphosis and spinal skeletal abnormalities with intrathoracic stomach: a link toward understanding its pathogenesis. *J Am Coll Surg, 208*, 562-9.

[8]   Stylopoulos N., Gazelle G.S., Rattner D.W. (2002) Paraesophageal hernias: operation or observation? *Ann Surg, 236*, 492-501.

[9]   Athanasakis H., Tzortzinis A., Tsiaoussis J., Vassilakis J.S., Xynos E. (2001) Laparoscopic repair of paraesophageal hernia. *Endoscopy, 33*, 590-4.

[10] Hashemi M., Peters J.H., DeMeester T.R., Huprich J.E., Quek M., Hagen J.A., Crookes P.F., Theisen J., DeMeester S.R., Sillin L.F., Bremner C.G. (2000) Laparoscopic repair of large type III hiatal hernia: objective followup reveals high recurrence rate. *J Am Coll Surg, 190*, 553-60.

[11] Lin E., Swafford V., Chadalavada R., Ramshow B.G., Smith C.D. (2004) Disparity between symptomatic and physiologic outcomes following esophageal lengthening procedures for antireflux surgery. *J Gastrointest Surg, 8*, 31-9.

[12] Mehta S., Boddy A., Rhodes M. (2006) Review of outcome after laparoscopic paraesophageal hiatal hernia repair. *Surg Lapar Endosc Percutan Tech, 16*, 301-6.

[13]Trus T.L., Bax T., Richardson W.S., Branum G.D., Mauren S.J., Swanstrom L.L., Hunter J.G. (1997) Complications of laparoscopic paraesophageal hernia repair. *J Gastrointest Surg, 1*, 221-228.

[14]Kemppainen E., Kiviluoto T. (2000) Fatal cardiac tamponade after emergency tension-free repair of a large paraesophageal hernia. *Surg Endosc, 14*, 593.

[15]Stadlhuber R.J., Sherif A.E., Mittal S.K., Fitzgibbons R.J. Jr., Brunt M.L., Hunter J.G., Demeester T.R., Swanstrom L.L., Daniel Smith C., Filipi C.J. (2009) Mesh complications after prosthetic reinforcement of hiatal closure: a 28-case series. *Surg Endosc, 23*, 1219-26.

[16]Johnson J.M., Carbonell A.M., Carmody B.J, Jamal M.K., Maher J.W., Kellum J.M., DeMaria E.J. (2006) Laparoscopic mesh hiatoplasty for paraesophageal hernias and fundoplications: a critical analysis og the available literature. *Surg Endosc, 20*, 362-6.

[17]Soricelli E., Basso N., Genco A., Cipriano M. (2009) Long-term results of hiatal hernia mesh repair and antireflux laparoscopic surgery. *Surg Endosc*, doi: 10.1007/s00464-009-0425-3.

[18]Kamolz T., Granderath FA., Bammer T., Pasiut M., Pointner R. (2002) Dysphagia and quality of life after laparoscopic Nissen fundoplication in patients with and without prosthetic reinforcement of the hiatal crura. *Surg Endosc, 16*, 572-7.

[19]Dally E., Falt G.L. (2004) Teflon pledget reinforced fundoplication causes symptomatic gastric and esophageal lumenal penetration. *Am J Surg, 187*, 226-9.

[20]Soper N.J., Dunnegan D. (1999) Anatomic fundoplication failure after laparoscopic antireflux surgery. *Ann Surg, 229*, 669-77.

[21]Watson D.I., Davies N., Devitt P.G., Jamieson G.G. (1999) Importance of dissection of the hernial sac in laparoscopic surgery for large hiatal hernias. *Arch Surg, 134*, 1069-73.

[22]Granderath F.A., Schweiger U.M., Pointner R. (2007) Laparoscopic antireflux surgery: Tailoring the hiatal closure to the size of hiatal surface area. *Surg Endosc, 21*, 542-8.

[23]Rathore M.A., Andrabi S.I., Bhatti M.I., Najfi S.M., McMurray A. (2007) Metaanalysis of recurrence after laparoscopic repair of paraesophageal hernia. *JSLS, 11*, 456-60.

[24]Hatch K.F., Daily M.F., Christensen B.J., Glasgow R.E. (2004) Failed fundoplications. *Am J Surg, 188*, 786-91.

[25] Granderath F.A., Granderath U.M., Pointner R. (2008) Laparoscopic revisional fundoplication with circular hiatal mesh prosthesis: The long-term results. *World J Surg, 32*, 999-1007.

[26] Granderath F.A., Kamolz T., Schweiger U.M., Pointner R. (2003) Laparoscopic refundoplication with prosthetic hiatal closure for recurrent hiatal hernia after primary failed antireflux surgery. *Arch Surg, 138*, 902-7.

[27] Basso N., De Leo A., Genco A. Rosato P., Rea S., Spaziani E., Primavera A. (2000) 360° laparoscopic fundoplication with tension-free hiatoplasty in the treatment of symptomatic gastroesophageal reflux disease. *Surg Endosc, 14*, 164-9.

[28] Huntington T.R. (1997) Laparoscopic mesh repair of the esophageal hiatus. *J Am Coll Surg, 184*, 399-401.

[29] Granderath F.A., Schweiger U.M., Kamolz T., Pasiut M., Haas C.F., Pointner R. (2002) Laparoscopic antireflux surgery with routine mesh-hiatoplasty in the treatment of gastroesophageal reflux disease. *J Gastrointest Surg, 6*, 347-353.

[30] Carlson M.A., Condon R.E., Ludwig K.A., Schulte W.J. (1998) Management of intrathoracic stomach with polypropylene mesh prosthesis reinforced transabdominal hiatus hernia repair. *J Am Coll Surg, 187*, 227-30.

[31] Rauth T., Poulose B., Nanney L., Holzman M. (2007) A comparative analysis of expanded polytetrafluoroethylene and small intestinal submucosa - Implications for patch repair in ventral herniorrhaphy *J Surg Res, 143*, 43-49.

[32] Oelschlager B.K., Barreca M., Chang L., Pellegrini C.A. (2003) The use of small intestine submucosa in the repair of paraesophageal hernias: initial observations of a new technique. Am J Surg,186, 4-8.

[33] Granderath F.A., Schweiger U.M., Kamolz T., Pointner R. (2005) Dysphagia after laparoscopic antireflux surgery: a problem of the hiatal closure more than a problem of the wrap. Surg Endosc, 19, 1439-46.

[34] Larusson H.J., Zingg U., Hahnloser D., Delport K., Seifert B., Oertli D. (2009) Predictive factors for morbidity and mortality in patients undergoing laparoscopic paraesophageal hernia repair: age, ASA score and operation type influence morbidity. *World J Surg, 33*, 980-5.

[35] Granderath F.A., Schweiger U.M., Kamolz T., Asche K.U., Pointner R. (2005) Laparoscopic Nissen fundoplication with prosthetic hiatal closure

reduces postoperative intrathoracic wrap herniation: Preliminary results of a prospective randomized functional and clinical study. *Arch Surg, 140*, 40-8.

[36] Willekes C.L., Edoga J.K., Freeza E.E. (1997) Laparoscopic repair of paraesophageal hernia. *Ann Surg, 225*, 31-38.

[37] Carlson M.A., Richards C.G., Frantzides C.T. (1999) Laparoscopic prosthetic reinforcement of hiatal herniorrhaphy. *Dig Surg, 16*, 407-10.

[38] Frantzides C.T., Madan A.K., Carlson M.A., Stavropoulos G.P. (2002) A prospective, randomized trial of laparoscopic polytetrafluoroethylene (PTFE) patch repair vs simple cruroplasty for large hiatal hernia. *Arch Surg, 137*, 649-52.

[39] Granderath F.A., Kamolz T., Schweiger U.M., Pointner R. (2002) Long-term follow-up after laparoscopic refundoplication for failed antireflux surgery: quality of life, symptomatic outcome, and patient satisfaction. J Gastrointest Surg, 6, 812-8.

[40] Champion J.K., Rock D. (2003) Laparoscopic mesh cruroplasty for large paraesophageal hernias. *Surg Endosc, 17*, 551-3.

[41] Gryska P.V., Vernon J.K. (2005) Tension-free repair of hiatal hernia during laparoscopic fundoplication: a ten-year experience. *Hernia, 9*, 150-5.

[42] Granderath F.A., Kamolz T., Schweiger U.M., Pointner R. (2006) Impact of laparoscopic nissen fundoplication with prosthetic hiatal closure on esophageal body motility: Results of a prospective randomized trial. *Arch Surg, 141*, 625-32.

[43] Kepenekci I. (2007) Laparoscopic fundoplication with prosthetic hiatal closure. *World J Surg, 31*, 2169-76.

[44] Zaninotto G., Portale G., Costantini M., Fiamingo P., Rampado S., Guirroli E., Nicoletti L., Ancona E. (2007) Objective follow-up after laparoscopic repair of large type III hiatal hernia. Assessment of safety and durability. *World J Surg, 31*, 2177-83.

[45] Lubezky N., Sagie B., Keidar A., Szold A. (2007) Prosthetic mesh repair of large and recurrent diaphragmatic hernias. *Surg Endosc 21*, 737-41.

[46] Jacobs M., Gomez E., Plasencia G., Lopez-Penalver C., Lujan H., Velarde D, Jessee T. (2007) Use of Surgisis mesh in laparoscopic repair of hiatal hernias. *Surg Laparosc Endosc Percutan Tech, 17*, 365-8.

[47]Lee E., Frisella M.M., Matthews B.D., Brunt L.M. (2007) Evaluation of acellular human dermis reinforcement of the crural closure in patients with difficult hiatal hernias. *Surg Endosc, 21*, 641-5.

[48]Hazebroek E.J., Ng A., Yong D.H., Berry H., Leibman S., Smith G.S. (2008) Evaluation of lightweight titanium-coated polypropylene mesh (TiMesh) for laparoscopic repair of large hiatal hernias. *Surg Endosc, 22*, 2428-32.

[49]Lee Y.K., James E., Bochkarev V., Vitamvas M., Oleynikov D. (2008) Long-term outcome of cruroplasty reinforcement with human acellular dermal matrix in large paraesophageal hiatal hernia. *J Gastrointest Surg, 12*, 811-5.

[50]Varga G., Cseke L., Kalmar K., Horvath O.P. (2008) Laparoscopic repair of large hiatal hernia with teres ligament: midterm follow-up. Surg Endosc, 22, 881-4.

[51]Zehetner J., Lipham J.C., Ayazi S., Oezcelik A., Abate E., Chen W., DeMeester S.R., Sohn H.J., Banki F., Hagen J.A., Dickey M., DeMeester T.R. (2009) A simplified technique for intrathoracic stomach laparoscopic fundoplication with Vicryl mesh and reinforcement. *Surg Endosc*, doi: 10.1007/s00464-009-0662-5.

[52]Müller-Stich B.P., Köninger J., Müller-Stich B.H., Schäfer F., Warschkow R., Mehrabi A., Gutt C.N. (2009) Laparoscopic mesh-augmented hiatoplasty as a method to treat gastroesophageal reflux without fundoplication: single-center experience with 306 consecutive patients. *Am J Surg, 198*, 17-24.

[53]Hazebroek E.J., Koak Y., Berry H., Leibman S., Smith G.S. (2009) Critical evaluation of a novel DualMesh repair for large hiatal hernias. *Surg Endosc, 23*, 193-6.

In: Reflux Disease: Causes, Symptoms and ...   ISBN: 978-1-61668-694-9
Editor: G. M. Esposito, pp. 127-139   © 2010 Nova Science Publishers, Inc.

Chapter V

THE MINIMALLY INVASIVE TREATMENT OF GASTROESOPHAGEAL REFLUX DISEASE

V. Shankaran, A. Baldea, R. J. Joehl and P. M. Fisichella[*]
Loyola University Medical Center, Chicago, Illinois, USA.

BRIEF HISTORY

Karl Rokitansky first identified a relation between gastric acid and esophageal pathology in the 19th century [1]. While other physicians studied esophageal ulcerations, Asher Winkelstein was the first one to define reflux esophagitis in 1934. He documented a series of patients suffering from chronic substernal pain, heartburn, and regurgitation with diffuse esophageal inflammation on esophagoscopy. All patients in his series achieved some symptomatic relief with antacid therapy consisting of alkalinized intragastric milk [2]. Even decades after his original work, Winkelstein's initial

---

[*] Correspondence concerning this article should be addressed to: Piero M. Fisichella, MD, Director Swallowing Center, Loyola University Medical Center, Department of Surgery, Stritch School of Medicine, 2160 South First Avenue - Room 3226. Maywood, IL 60153. Phone: (708) 327-2236; Fax: (708) 327-3492.

description and findings of gastroesophageal reflux disease (GERD) remain largely unchanged.

EPIDEMIOLOGY

Over the past few decades, GERD has become increasingly diagnosed and treated. GERD currently accounts for about 75% of esophageal disease. Approximately 20% of people in the United States suffer from GERD and 30-40% of patients regularly complain of symptoms typically associated with GERD [3]. Due to the high prevalence of GERD, numerous studies have been performed to determine its causative factors. The correlation of obesity to reflux symptoms and GERD has been object of intense scrutiny. Obesity rates are increasing in the United States; approximately 33% of the adult population in this country is classified as obese, representing a two- to three-fold increase over the past 50 years [4]. The rates of GERD are also rapidly increasing, with its worldwide prevalence increasing by 4% yearly. Obese patients are 2.5 times more likely to have GERD symptoms or esophageal erosions as normal-weight patients, the two are presumptively closely linked [5]. It has been hypothesized that increased visceral adipose tissue in obese patients results in higher intra-gastric pressure. Intra-abdominal pressure is also increased by congestive heart failure and hypertension, both of which occur more commonly in the obese population. It has also been suggested that increased lipolysis and free fatty acids associated with increased visceral adipose tissue may induce the release of pro-inflammatory cytokines that reduce lower esophageal sphincter (LES) pressure. Both increased intra-abdominal pressure and decreased LES pressure decrease LES competence, thereby increasing the risk for GERD in the obese population [6]. Moreover, body mass index (BMI), an index relating body weight to height, has been shown to be an independent risk factor for hiatal hernia, which itself is a risk factor for GERD.

In addition to obesity, certain foods are thought to induce GERD and reflux symptoms. A study by Shapiro et al. identified an increase in reflux symptoms with cholesterol and saturated fat consumption and a decrease with high fiber intake [7]. Similarly, several studies have demonstrated a decrease in LES pressure with ingestion of fats and chocolate [8,9]. Often, simple lifestyle modifications including weight loss, dietary modification, and tobacco cessation may significantly reduce GERD or reflux symptoms, and therefore remain the first-line treatment for GERD.

DIAGNOSTIC STUDIES

The diagnosis of GERD and its associated anatomic anomalies (hiatal hernias, strictures, diverticula) is best achieved by: a symptomatic assessment, ambulatory pH monitoring, esophageal manometry, upper endoscopy, and upper gastrointestinal series. This thorough evaluation objectively confirms the presence of GERD, severity of reflux, degree of mucosal damage, correlation between symptoms and reflux events, identifies any anatomic abnormalities that may contribute to esophageal dysfunction, and rules out other organic causes that might be responsible for the clinical symptoms.

The diagnosis of GERD may not be made on symptoms alone, though the presence of symptoms may raise clinical suspicion enough to warrant further testing. Symptoms may be classified into typical or atypical; heartburn and regurgitation are typical symptoms, while cough, hoarseness, and chest pain are considered atypical symptoms. This classification is important as it is predictive of response to both medical and surgical intervention for GERD [10,11]. An Australian study from 2008 followed 155 patients with positive ambulatory pH results who underwent antireflux surgery [12]. The patients in which reflux events correlated with typical symptoms as opposed to those with atypical or no symptoms attained better relief and were more satisfied following antireflux surgery. Moreover, while symptoms alone may point to the diagnosis of GERD, they are not a reliable indicator of the presence of disease. A 2001 study of 822 patients demonstrated that only 70% of patients with complaints of typical reflux symptoms demonstrated objective gastroesophageal reflux on ambulatory pH monitoring [10].

Today, the gold standard test for the diagnosis of GERD is ambulatory esophageal pH monitoring. Gastric pH detection was introduced in the late 19th century by Reichman, but the first measurement of esophageal pH was not performed until 1958, when Tuttle and Grossman used a gastric pH probe to determine the pH of the esophagus along different positions. The current practice of measurement was described by Johnson and DeMeester in 1974. A pH sensor is placed 5 cm above the lower esophageal sphincter and the number and length of episodes in which the pH is less than 4 are tabulated

[13]. In addition to establishing a definitive diagnosis, ambulatory pH monitoring correlates the chronology of symptoms with reflux events. Ambulatory pH monitoring has a sensitivity and specificity of 92%, thereby making it the most reliable test for the diagnosis of GERD [14].

Esophageal manometry is a test of the quality of esophageal peristalsis. Manometry provides a more thorough evaluation of the esophagus as it can diagnose esophageal motility disorders. Additionally, it provides data about lower esophageal sphincter function (resting pressure, length, relaxation) that facilitates proper positioning of the pH probe [13].

Upper endoscopy is useful to diagnose complications of GERD such as esophagitis, Barrett's esophagus, or strictures. It is often one of the first tests performed on patients with complaints of typical reflux symptoms. Endoscopy alone or in conjunction with symptomatic assessment, however, is not adequate for diagnosis of GERD, as mucosal changes are absent in 50% of GERD patients. In addition, it has been shown that the interobserver agreement among pathologists about lower grades of esophagitis is poor [15].

An upper gastrointestinal series may suggest GERD, but diagnosis cannot be based on the results of this test. It is a test performed to determine anatomic abnormalities, such as hiatal hernia or esophageal stricture, which may contribute to patient symptoms. The anatomic information gleaned from this test may also help in operative planning.

The definitive diagnosis and evaluation of GERD requires a series of tests detailed as above. While each test has its individual attributes and utilities, the collective data derives from these tests best allows for the diagnosis and optimal management of GERD.

MEDICAL TREATMENT

The true prevalence of GERD is unknown as many patients seldom seek care from a physician; however, GERD is broadly accepted as the most common esophageal disease in the United States. The first-line treatment is lifestyle modification, with weight loss and an exercise regimen as the cornerstones. Patients are advised to eat frequent small meals during the day to avoid gastric distension and to avoid spicy/fatty foods and chocolate. Patients are also advised to eat the last meal at least 2 hours before going to bed and elevating the head of bed to minimize the effects of gravity. Unfortunately these lifestyle modifications are difficult for some patients to adhere to; moreover, they rarely fully alleviate symptoms [16].

Though controlled weight loss and moderate activity have both been shown to reduce GERD and its associated symptoms, lifestyle changes alone are rarely adequate treatment of GERD. Medical therapies for GERD have been used for centuries. Earlier regimens included the use of herbal remedies including cannabis and cocaine. In the 20th century, however, milk and antacids became accepted therapeutics [1]. Medical treatment has since continued to evolve, and since the development of H_2 receptor antagonists in the 1970s and proton pump inhibitors (PPIs) in the 1990s, medical therapy has become an effective adjunct to lifestyle changes. In general, H_2 receptor antagonists are prescribed for patients with mild esophagitis and mild reflux symptoms. Since were first introduced in the early-1990s, however, PPIs have become the mainstay of medical therapy for GERD. The majority of patients with symptomatic GERD, particularly those with typical symptoms, gain some relief with the use of a PPI. In fact, esophageal healing is noted in 80-90% of patients with esophagitis who regularly use PPIs; however, the symptoms and esophageal inflammation usually recur soon after discontinuation of medications [17,18]. Because of their efficacy in relieving GERD and its symptoms, the use of PPIs has risen considerably and overuse has become a problem. As with all medications, PPIs are not without side effects. Patients commonly complain of headaches, nausea, abdominal pain, and flatulence. While these side-effects are generally innocuous and self-limited, numerous complications of long-term PPI use have been reported. Chronic PPI use has been shown to cause calcium malabsorption in the gastrointestinal tract by altering the optimal pH for absorption. A study by Yang et al demonstrated a significant increase in the rate of hip fractures in patients using chronic PPI therapy (adjusted odds ratio 1.44), a finding believed to be due to decreased calcium absorption and decreased bone resorption due to inhibition of osteoclasts proton pumps by PPI therapy [19]. Chronic acid suppression due to PPI use has also been implicated in increased rates of infective diarrhea, including *Clostridium difficile* colitis [20]. Recent studies have also demonstrated a decrease in the efficacy of anti-platelet medications, specifically clopidogrel, in PPI users. A study by Ho et al of 8205 patients hospitalized for acute coronary syndrome noted a statistically significant increase in rehospitalization and death rates in the group of patients using proton pump inhibitors [21]. While more studies are needed to fully determine the potential detriments of chronic PPI use, in higher risk populations caution should be used in prescribing long-term therapy with PPIs.

SURGICAL TREATMENT

Indications for Surgery

Laparoscopic antireflux surgery is indicated in several groups of patients, including young patients who require chronic PPI use to control symptoms, patients with regurgitation despite medical therapy, patients with respiratory symptoms (cough or aspiration) when GERD is also present, and in patients with Barrett's esophagus. Campos et al. demonstrated that an abnormal ambulatory pH monitoring, together with a good response to acid suppression therapy and the presence of typical symptoms, such as heartburn and regurgitation, predict a successful outcome of laparoscopic antireflux surgery [22]. Similarly, Morgenthal et al. identified preoperative predictors of success in a 312 patients who underwent laparoscopic Nissen fundoplication between 1992 and 1995. Response and lack of response to anti-reflux medications were associated with 77% and 56% success rates respectively ($p = 0.035$). Eighty five percent of patients with typical symptoms had a successful outcome, compared to only 41% with atypical symptoms ($p < 0.001$) [23]. Preoperative Body Mass Index (BMI) greater than 35 kg/m^2) was associated with failure ($p = 0.036$), while a BMI of 30-34.9 kg/m^2 was not. These studies helped to predictably identify which patients will fare well after surgery, and explicitly stressed that an excellent outcome is based upon an objective diagnosis of GERD, rather than a diagnosis merely based on symptoms. Several studies have demonstrated that antireflux surgery prevents the development of Barrett's metaplasia in patients with GERD. A study by Oelschlager et al demonstrated regression or elimination of Barrett's esophagus in 55% of patients with short-segment disease (<3cm). As medical therapy alone will only prevent progression of Barrett's esophagus and progression will occur if therapy is stopped, surgery is a valuable treatment modality in patients with Barrett's changes [24].

Pre-operative Evaluation

Prior to undergoing surgery, all candidates should receive a full medical evaluation and undergo a full battery of testing including symptomatic assessment, esophagoscopy, upper GI series, ambulatory pH monitoring, and esophageal manometry.

The decision of whether to perform a partial or total fundoplication based on esophageal function testing, the so-called "tailored approach", has been extensively studied. Horvath et al. and Oleynikov et al. showed that the laparoscopic partial fundoplication was effective in controlling reflux by pH monitoring in less than half of the patients [25,26]. A randomized controlled trial of 106 patients assigned to laparoscopic total or partial fundoplication, regardless of preoperative esophageal dysmotility, demonstrated no difference in the incidence of postoperative dysphagia [27]. In 2001, Fibbe et al achieved similar conclusions in a controlled trial in which 200 patients were stratified according to presence or absence of esophageal dysmotility and randomized to either 360 degree (Nissen) or 270 degree (Toupet) fundoplication [28]. In this study, the authors showed that clinical outcome and reflux recurrence were similar (21% vs. 14%) in patients with and without dysmotility. The authors concluded that laparoscopic partial fundoplication was less effective than total fundoplication for treatment of reflux, and compared with a partial (240 degrees) fundoplication, a total (360 degree) fundoplication was not followed by more dysphagia, even when esophageal peristalsis was weak.

Today, a Nissen fundoplication (360 degree) is the procedure of choice except in those patients with GERD who demonstrate absent esophageal peristalsis on manometric testing, such as in patients with scleroderma for which, a partial (240 to 280 degree) fundoplication is performed.

Long-term Results of Laparoscopic Antireflux Surgery

The initial results of laparoscopic fundoplication obtained in the early 1990s indicated that the operation was as effective in controlling gastroesophageal reflux and its symptoms as the traditional open fundoplication. Early studies; however, reported "failure rates" nearing 30% with a significant number of patients reporting prolonged dysphagia. Patient satisfaction following surgery has risen significantly in the past decade to approximately 86-93% and the major complication rate has decreased to less than 5%. In retrospect, many of the poorer outcomes from the early 1990s have been attributed to technical inexperience [18,19].

As the learning curve progressed during the late 1990s, several studies analyzed the technical factors involved in the complications following laparoscopic fundoplication. In 1998, Soper, et al. described the incidence, precipitating factors, and management of these early technical failures of laparoscopic fundoplication [30]. In a group of 290 patients that underwent laparoscopic Nissen fundoplication by a single surgeon over a 6-year period, anatomic failure (defined as displacement or disruption/slippage of the fundoplication) was noted in 7% of the cases, with the majority in patients who had their procedure early in the learning curve. The authors noted that early on (the first 53 patients) the diaphragmatic crura were closed only in the presence of large hiatal hernias. Of the 20 failures in 290 cases, intrathoracic wrap migration was the most common cause of failure (13 patients, or 65%). Subsequent multivariate analysis demonstrated that four factors correlated with anatomic failure of the fundoplication: early experience, early postoperative vomiting, presence of diaphragmatic stressors, such as mediastinal adhesions, and hiatal hernia bigger than 3 cm. The authors concluded that full esophageal mobilization and meticulous closure of the diaphragmatic crura posterior to the esophagus should minimize anatomic functional failure after laparoscopic antireflux surgery.

In the early 2000s, reports from Europe and United States on the medium-term results (5-year) of the laparoscopic Nissen fundoplication in the control of GERD confirmed that reflux could be controlled effectively and for many years. In 2003, Anvari and Allen reported the 5-year comprehensive follow-up of 181 patients after undergoing laparoscopic fundoplication [31]. They reported that laparoscopic fundoplication was associated with a significant increase in lower esophageal sphincter pressure, a significant drop in duration of acid reflux in 24 hours, and a lower symptom score, 6, 24, and 60 months after surgery when compared with preoperative values. Twenty-one patients (12%) experienced recurrence of symptoms, but only six were reoperated. Patient satisfaction with surgery remained high, at 86%, after 5 years. Approximately 12% of patients resumed H_2 blockers or PPI but only 5% of all patients were found to have abnormal reflux score. In 2005, a large retrospective French multicenter study of 1340 patients with GERD undergoing fundoplication (711 patients underwent complete fundoplication,

559 underwent partial posterior fundoplication, and 70 underwent partial anterior fundoplication) between January 1992 and December 1998 reported a dysphagia rate of 5%, reoperation rate of 4.4%, and a recurrence rate of 10% five years following surgery [32].

Only few studies have a follow-up longer than 5 years. Dallemagne et al. followed for 10 years 100 consecutive patients on whom he operated in 1993 (Nissen fundoplication was performed in 68 patients, and partial posterior fundoplication was performed in 32 patients) and showed that at 5 years, 93% of the patients were free of symptoms and that at 10 years, 89% of the patients still were free of significant reflux (93% after Nissen, 82% after Toupet) [33]. Four patients underwent reoperation: one patient for persistent dysphagia and three patients for recurrent symptoms. In addition, at 5 years, 9 patients resumed antisecretory medications and, at 10 years, only 6 additional patients resumed antisecretory medications.

In 2008, Oelschlager et al. demonstrated that laparoscopic antireflux surgery improved heartburn and regurgitation in 90% and 92% of patients respectively in a study of 288 patients. This population also had a low incidence of new onset dysphagia (2%) or reoperation (3%) [34]. In addition, 66 patients (23%) resumed PPI.

In order to critically assess 10 years outcomes, Dallemagne published his results on 100 consecutive patients after complete and partial fundoplication. He reported a 90% rate of symptomatic control of reflux symptoms at 5 and 10 years with less than 10% of patients using antiacid medications at 10 years; only one patient in this series needed reintervention for persistent dysphagia [33]. Similar results have been reported by Zaninotto et al in a study of 399 patients for an average of 8 years following antireflux surgery. The study reported an 86% success rate of laparoscopic antireflux surgery, with only 3% of patients in the study requiring treatment (either endoscopically or with surgical revision) for persistent dysphagia. Approximately 21% of the study patients required PPIs 8 years post-operatively, but only 4% of study patients revealed endoscopic or manometric evidence of significant reflux [35]. Both of these studies support laparoscopic fundoplication as an effective and durable treatment for GERD.

CONCLUSIONS

Since the early 1990s, both improvements in medical therapy for GERD and the introduction of laparoscopic antireflux surgery have greatly changed the treatment of GERD. Today the laparoscopic Nissen fundoplication is considered the standard surgical approach for patients with GERD. Long-term results of this operation are excellent, provided that the technical element of the operation are performed carefully, and that characteristics of patients that are likely to benefit from laparoscopic antireflux surgery are properly identified preoperatively.

REFERENCES

[1] Modlin IM, Moss SF, Kidd M, Lye KD. Gastroesophageal reflux disease: then and now. *J Clin Gastroenterol* 2004; 38:390-402.

[2] Winkelstein A. Peptic Esophagitis. *Am J Med Sci* 1933; 104:906-09.

[3] Wang C, Hunt RH. Medical management of gastroesophageal reflux disease. *Gastroenterol Clin North Am* 2008; 37:879-99, ix.

[4] Fass R. The pathophysiological mechanisms of GERD in the obese patient. *Dig Dis Sci* 2008; 53:2300-6.

[5] Pandolfino JE, Kwiatek MA, Kahrilas PJ. The pathophysiologic basis for epidemiologic trends in gastroesophageal reflux disease. *Gastroenterol Clin North Am* 2008; 37:827-43, viii.

[6] Fisichella PM, Patti MG. Gastroesophageal reflux disease and morbid obesity: is there a relation? *World J Surg* 2009; 33:2034-8.

[7] Shapiro M, Green C, Bautista JM, et al. Assessment of dietary nutrients that influence perception of intra-oesophageal acid reflux events in patients with gastro-oesophageal reflux disease. *Aliment Pharmacol Ther* 2007; 25:93-101.

[8] Dore MP, Maragkoudakis E, Fraley K, et al. Diet, lifestyle and gender in gastro-esophageal reflux disease. *Dig Dis Sci* 2008; 53:2027-32.

[9] Murphy DW, Castell DO. Chocolate and heartburn: evidence of increased esophageal acid exposure after chocolate ingestion. *Am J Gastroenterol* 1988; 83:633-6.

[10]Patti MG, Diener U, Tamburini A, et al. Role of esophageal function tests in diagnosis of gastroesophageal reflux disease. *Dig Dis Sci* 2001; 46:597-602.

[11]Aanen MC, Bredenoord AJ, Numans ME, et al. Reproducibility of symptom association analysis in ambulatory reflux monitoring. *Am J Gastroenterol* 2008; 103:2200-8.

[12]Thompson SK, Cai W, Jamieson GG, et al. Recurrent symptoms after fundoplication with a negative pH study--recurrent reflux or functional heartburn? *J Gastrointest Surg* 2009; 13:54-60.

[13]Herbella FA, Nipominick I, Patti MG. From sponges to capsules. The history of esophageal pH monitoring. *Dis Esophagus* 2009; 22:99-103.

[14]Fuchs KH, DeMeester TR, Albertucci M. Specificity and sensitivity of objective diagnosis of gastroesophageal reflux disease. *Surgery* 1987; 102:575-80.

[15]Bytzer P, Havelund T, Hansen JM. Interobserver variation in the endoscopic diagnosis of reflux esophagitis. *Scand J Gastroenterol* 1993; 28:119-25.

[16]Festi D, Scaioli E, Baldi F, et al. Body weight, lifestyle, dietary habits and gastroesophageal reflux disease. *World J Gastroenterol* 2009; 15:1690-701.

[17]Grant AM, Wileman SM, Ramsay CR, et al. Minimal access surgery compared with medical management for chronic gastro-oesophageal reflux disease: UK collaborative randomised trial. *BMJ* 2008; 337:a2664.

[18]Vakil N. Review article: the role of surgery in gastro-oesophageal reflux disease. *Aliment Pharmacol Ther* 2007; 25:1365-72.

[19]Yang YX, Lewis JD, Epstein S, Metz DC. Long-term proton pump inhibitor therapy and risk of hip fracture. *JAMA* 2006; 296:2947-53.

[20]Ali T, Roberts DN, Tierney WM. Long-term safety concerns with proton pump inhibitors. *Am J Med* 2009; 122:896-903.

[21]Ho PM, Maddox TM, Wang L, et al. Risk of adverse outcomes associated with concomitant use of clopidogrel and proton pump inhibitors following acute coronary syndrome. *JAMA* 2009; 301:937-44.

[22]Campos GM, Peters JH, DeMeester TR, et al. Multivariate analysis of factors predicting outcome after laparoscopic Nissen fundoplication. *J Gastrointest Surg* 1999; 3:292-300.

[23] Morgenthal CB, Lin E, Shane MD, et al. Who will fail laparoscopic Nissen fundoplication? Preoperative prediction of long-term outcomes. *Surg Endosc* 2007; 21:1978-84.

[24] Oelschlager BK, Barreca M, Chang L, et al. Clinical and pathologic response of Barrett's esophagus to laparoscopic antireflux surgery. *Ann Surg* 2003; 238:458-64; discussion 64-6.

[25] Oleynikov D, Eubanks TR, Oelschlager BK, Pellegrini CA. Total fundoplication is the operation of choice for patients with gastroesophageal reflux and defective peristalsis. *Surg Endosc* 2002; 16:909-13.

[26] Horvath KD, Jobe BA, Herron DM, Swanstrom LL. Laparoscopic Toupet fundoplication is an inadequate procedure for patients with severe reflux disease. *J Gastrointest Surg* 1999; 3:583-91.

[27] Rydberg L, Ruth M, Abrahamsson H, Lundell L. Tailoring antireflux surgery: A randomized clinical trial. *World J Surg* 1999; 23:612-8.

[28] Fibbe C, Layer P, Keller J, et al. Esophageal motility in reflux disease before and after fundoplication: a prospective, randomized, clinical, and manometric study. *Gastroenterology* 2001; 121:5-14.

[29] Pohl D, Eubanks TR, Omelanczuk PE, Pellegrini CA. Management and outcome of complications after laparoscopic antireflux operations. *Arch Surg* 2001; 136:399-404.

[30] Soper NJ, Dunnegan D. Anatomic fundoplication failure after laparoscopic antireflux surgery. *Ann Surg* 1999; 229:669-76; discussion 76-7.

[31] Anvari M, Allen C. Five-year comprehensive outcomes evaluation in 181 patients after laparoscopic Nissen fundoplication. *J Am Coll Surg* 2003; 196:51-7; discussion 57-8; author reply 58-9.

[32] Pessaux P, Arnaud JP, Delattre JF, et al. Laparoscopic antireflux surgery: five-year results and beyond in 1340 patients. *Arch Surg* 2005; 140:946-51.

[33] Dallemagne B, Weerts J, Markiewicz S, et al. Clinical results of laparoscopic fundoplication at ten years after surgery. *Surg Endosc* 2006; 20:159-65.

[34] Oelschlager BK, Quiroga E, Parra JD, et al. Long-term outcomes after laparoscopic antireflux surgery. *Am J Gastroenterol* 2008; 103:280-7; quiz 88.

[35]Zaninotto G, Portale G, Costantini M, et al. Long-term results (6-10 years) of laparoscopic fundoplication. *J Gastrointest Surg* 2007; 11:1138-45.

In: Reflux Disease: Causes, Symptoms and ...   ISBN: 978-1-61668-694-9
Editor: G. M. Esposito, pp. 141-155   © 2010 Nova Science Publishers, Inc.

Chapter VI

Anatomy and Physiology of the Esophagus

C.S. Davis, R.J. Joehl and P.M. Fisichella[*]
Loyola University Medical Center, Chicago, Illinois

Abstract

The normal physiology of the esophagus is complex and not completely understood. Recent evolution of diagnostic technology in the field of esophageal motility testing has helped the clinician in better understanding the normal physiology of the esophagus and in the management of patients with esophageal disorders. The purpose of this chapter is to give a comprehensive review of the normal anatomy of the esophagus with particular interest to its function, in light of the recent anatomic and physiologic findings obtained by high-resolution esophageal impedance manometry. The Authors describe the anatomic makeup of each area of the esophagus: the upper esophageal sphincter (UES), the body, and the lower esophageal sphincter (LES). Further emphasis is placed on the physiologic function of each anatomic area,

[*] Corresponding Author: Piero M. Fisichella, MD, Director Swallowing Center, Loyola University Medical Center, Department of Surgery, Stritch School of Medicine, 2160 South First Avenue - Room 3226., Maywood, IL 60153, Phone: (708) 327-2236, Fax: (708) 327-3492

and the mechanisms of the coordinated motor activity that ultimately results in the passage of food from the pharynx into the stomach.

INTRODUCTION

Beginning at the level of the 6th cervical vertebra and ending at the level of the 11th thoracic vertebra, the esophagus is a neuromuscular tube comprised of striated muscle proximally, smooth muscle distally, and a myenteric plexus of nerves throughout. Understanding of both the anatomic and functional divisions of this neuromuscular organ is essential. As such, three primary anatomic areas can be delineated: the cervical esophagus, the thoracic esophagus, and the abdominal esophagus. Likewise, there are three functional areas, those being the UES, the esophageal body, and the LES. Proper coordination of the esophageal sphincters with the forward propulsion of a swallowed bolus that occurs in the esophageal body is critical to both airway protection and to mitigate reflux of gastric contents back into the esophagus. Dysfunctional coordination at any level may result in pathologic consequences, for which diagnosis by esophageal motility testing may aid in subsequent treatment decisions.

UPPER ESOPHAGEAL SPHINCTER

The first functional division of the esophagus, the UES, is high-pressure zone (100-140 mmHg), 2 to 4 centimeters in length, found at the level of the 6th to 7th cervical vertebrae [1]. Located between the pharynx and cervical esophagus, the physiologic role of the UES is to protect against reflux of gastric contents into the airways, as well as to prevent the entrance of air into the esophagus as a result of negative thoracic pressures [2, 4]. Embryologically derived from branchial cleft cells, the striated musculature of the UES consists of the cricopharyngeus (CP) muscle, the inferior constrictors of the pharynx, and the cervical esophagus. The most prominent muscular component of the UES, the CP, is comprised of a non-parallel arrangement of mostly slow-twitch (type 1, oxidative) and also fast-twitch (type 2, glycolytic) muscle fibers, allowing for maintenance of a constant basal tone, or resting pressure, as well as a rapid response to belching or swallowing [2, 38, 39].

Motor innervation to the CP and the rest of the UES is derived from the nucleus ambiguous (NA) in the brain stem, communicating to the CP via the pharyngo-esophageal and superior laryngeal nerves [4]. Although historically conjectural, there does appear to be minor functional innervation from the recurrent laryngeal nerve, whereby recurrent laryngeal nerve paresis may be associated with swallowing dysfunction. [3] Finally, sensory innervation to the UES is contributed by the glossopharyngeal nerve and cervical sympathetics.

Structurally, the UES is slit-like, with greater pressures generated in the anterior-posterior axis (100 mmHg) than laterally (50 mmHg) [4]. The high-pressure zone of the UES is distinguished by a peak in the high-pressure zone corresponding to the posterior surface of the cricoid cartilage and a decline in pressure distally that corresponds to the CP [1,2]. At rest, overall tone is likely a manifestation of both tonic muscular contraction and passive elastic forces (**Fig. 1**) [5].

The functionality of the UES is central to protecting the trachiobronchial tree from inadvertent passage of food, saliva, and gatric refluxate. Basal tone is primarily responsible for the latter, as the UES is the last barrier to aspiration of gastric contents. This phenomenon is demonstrated by a reflex increase of UES pressure with increased intraluminal distension, which may or may not as well be augmented by decreased intraluminal pH [6-8]. Nevertheless, patients with respiratory symptoms from aspiration of gastric contents often have associated esophageal motor disorders, a component of which may be a hypotensive UES. Additional protection of the tracheobronchial tree occurs during swallowing, the mechanics of which are highly coordinated. Swallowing in humans can be voluntary or involuntary [9]. In either case, the cricoid and hyoid bone are displaced upward and anteriorly by the mylohyoid, styloglossus, and hyoglossus muscles, thus propelling the bolus into the pharynx. At the same time, the soft palate is pulled upward, closing the posterior nares. The larynx itself is closed off by the backward motion of the epiglottis, which is directly responsible for the prevention of food passing into the tracheobronchial tree. As part of this complex reflex mechanism, respiration temporarily stops, the UES relaxes, the suprahyoid muscles contract, and the esophageal inlet opens [9]. The UES pressure is then immediately restored once the bolus reaches the cervical esophagus. (**Fig. 1**)

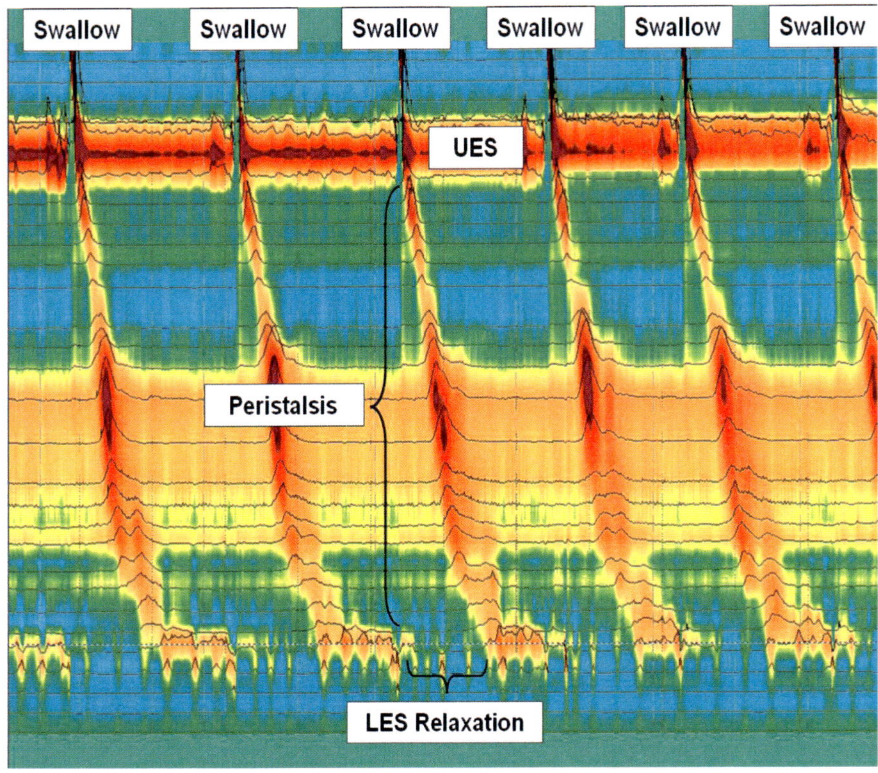

Figure 1. Normal sequence of swallowing during high-resolution esophageal manometry; both the UES and the LES relax after swallowing, while peristalsis is initiated once the bolus enters the esophagus. Then the LES closes after the bolus has entered into the stomach. Note that the UES and the LES are tonically contracted at rest.

ESOPHAGEAL BODY

The esophageal body is a neuromuscular tube whose primary function is peristalsis (**Fig. 1**); dysfunction of which may lead to disease. Excluding the UES and LES, the esophageal body is 18 to 22 cm in length. Measured from the incisors, the upper extent begins at approximately 18 cm, ending at 37 cm in women (range 22 to 41 cm) and 40 cm in men (range 26 to 50 cm) [9]. Unlike most of the rest of the gastrointestinal tract, the esophagus has no serosa, though the mucosa, submucosa, and muscularis propria are preserved.

The strength layer of the esophageal wall is the submucosa, with its elastic and fibrous tissue components [35]. The muscle fibers of the muscularis propria are arranged in outer longitudinal and inner circular layers, and share their muscular presence with the muscularis mucosa, which is a longitudinal component of muscular fibers between the muscularis propria and mucosa. Smooth muscle predominates at the level of the mid- and inferior esophagus, gradually taking the place of striated muscle that predominates in the upper one-third to upper half of the esophagus. Another distinguishing feature of the esophageal body is its intrinsic nervous system, **comprised of Meissner's** plexus and the myenteric plexus of Auerbach. These plexuses are found between the longitudinal and circular muscle layers, and between the circular muscle layer and muscularis mucosa, respectively. The myenteric plexus itself has both excitatory and inhibitory neurons. Here, excitatory neurons function through cholinergic receptors to control the longitudinal and circular muscle layers, and inhibitory neurons function through non-adrenergic, non-cholinergic neurotransmitters such as nitric oxide (NO) and vasoactive intestinal peptide (VIP) [9,31]. In concert with vagal innervation, the intrinsic nervous system establishes coordination of striated and smooth muscle activity. Specifically, vagal stimuli, by way of the recurrent laryngeal nerve, originate in the medulla and directly control striated muscle activity through acetylcholine-mediated excitatory signaling [9]. Vagal afferents also synapse directly on the neurons of the intramural plexuses to establish esophageal muscular control, which is also intrinsically mediated by the myenteric plexus independent of vagal stimulation. In the resting state, the esophageal body is devoid of motor activity [31].

Peristalsis in the esophageal body is classified as primary, secondary, or tertiary. *Primary peristalsis* is initiated by swallowing, and once a bolus has passed through the UES, the wave of contraction moves caudad toward the stomach (Fig. 1). The primary peristaltic wave proceeds distally at approximately 3-4 cm/second, peaking in amplitude at 60 to 140 mmHg as measured at the distal esophagus [36]. *Secondary peristalsis* is triggered locally (without central stimulation) by contents that remain in the esophageal body from incomplete clearance during primary peristalsis or by reflux of gastric contents [4]. Secondary peristaltic waves move distally from their site of origination. *Tertiary peristalsis* is pathologic and represents a series of non-propulsive contractions, which are usually found in patients with primary esophageal motility disorders [37]. In addition, when swallows rapidly follow one another by less than 5 seconds, peristalsis is temporarily inhibited by neural discharges from the central swallowing center, a phenomenon referred to as "*deglutitive inhibition*" [4]. **The accumulated bolus is then cleared by a** large single wave of peristalsis once the rapid sequence of swallowing has ceased.

Disruption of the normal peristaltic activity in the esophageal body can have numerous pathologic outcomes. Improper clearance of gastric refluxate is often attributable to impoverished peristaltic quality. Hypotensive peristalsis is one such phenomenon that may result in incomplete volume clearance [22]. *Ineffective esophageal peristalsis* is a term that refers to both hypotensive peristalsis (distal esophageal amplitude of less than 30 mmHg) and/or more than 30% simultaneous waves (**Fig. 2**) [23,24]. Such a condition may be associated with poor volume clearance, as well as with more proximal gastroesophageal reflux, whereby clearance of acidic content is delayed in both the distal and proximal esophagus. Ineffectiveness of peristalsis has also been associated with respiratory symptomatology secondary to airway aspiration **of gastric contents. Furthermore, Barrett's esophag**us is associated with impairment in peristalsis, presumably secondary to inflammatory changes induced by chronic exposure to acid and alkaline reflux.

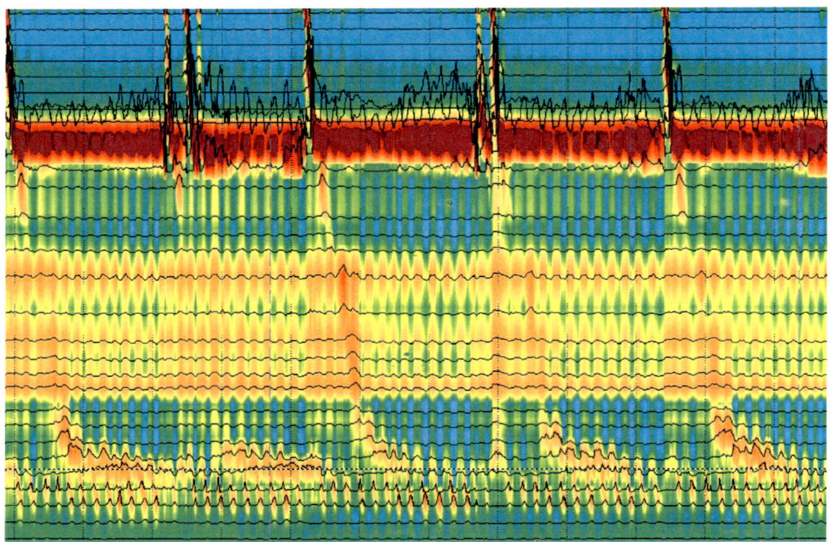

Figure 2. Ineffective esophageal peristalsis; high-resolution esophageal manometry shows hypotensive peristalsis (distal esophageal amplitude of less than 30 mmHg).

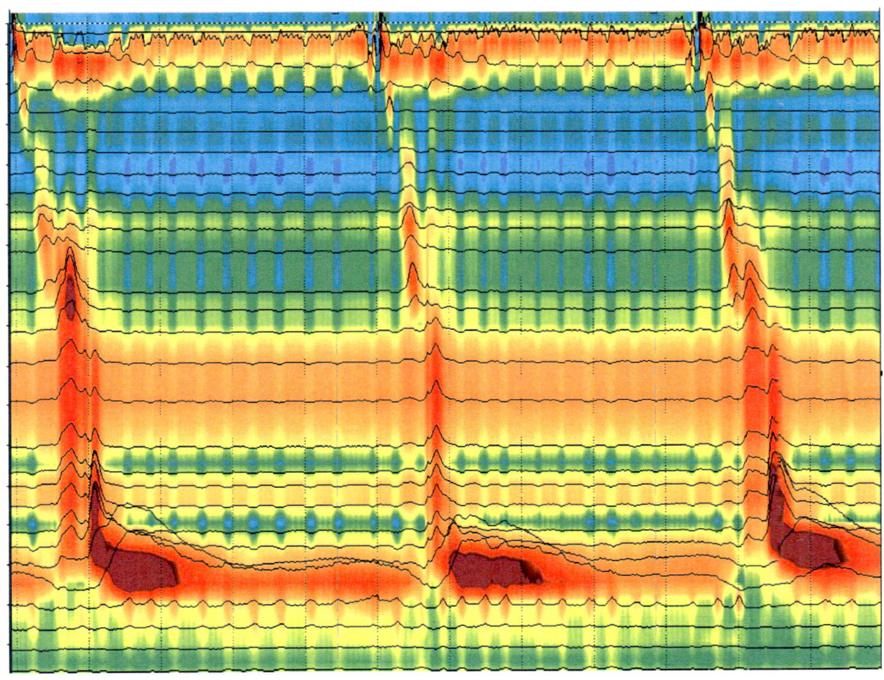

Figure 3. Achalasia; high-resolution esophageal manometry shows a hypertensive LES that partially relaxes after swallowing. Peristalsis is absent and only simultaneous "mirror images" waves can be appreciated.

Impairment of esophageal motility is classified into specific subsets of motility disorders. The *primary esophageal motility disorders* is one such subset, of which includes achalasia, hypertensive LES, diffuse esophageal spasm (DES), and nutcracker esophagus. In achalasia, the LES fails to relax with swallowing and peristalsis is absent (**Fig 3**). In hypertensive LES, peristalsis is preserved, while the hypertensive LES (>14 mmHg) relaxes appropriately with swallowing. In DES, diagnostic criteria require simultaneous contractions in greater than 10% of wet swallows, as well a mean amplitude of simultaneous contractions greater than 30 mmHg [26]. In nutcracker esophagus, the esophagus is subjected to high amplitude peristaltic contractions that may last longer than six seconds. Spechler and Castell propose that the manometric diagnosis of nutcracker esophagus be a mean peristaltic wave amplitude after 10 swallows of greater than 180 mmHg, as measured at the distal esophagus (**Fig 4**) [26]. Another subset of abnormal esophageal function is described as *nonspecific esophageal motility disorders* (NEMD), which, as demonstrated by esophageal manometry, are marked by low amplitude peristalsis and abnormal morphology (triple peaks and simultaneous contractions) of peristaltic waves. Additionally, gastroesophageal reflux disease (GERD) appears to have an intricate association with abnormalities of peristalsis. NEMD may in fact be responsible for symptomatic GERD as well as worsening its effects via inefficient clearance of gastric refluxate [23].

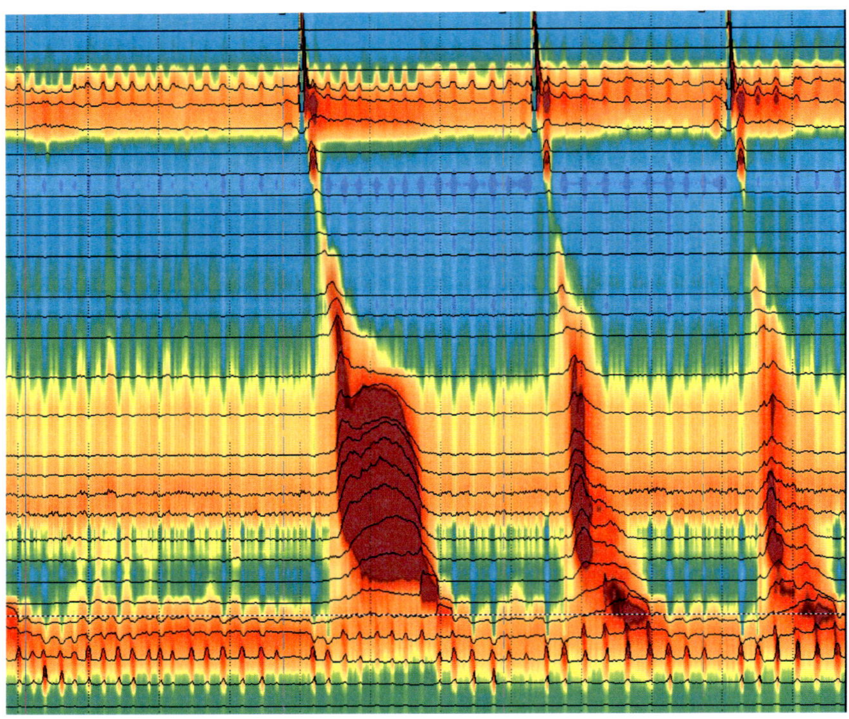

Figure 4. Nutcracker esophagus and esophageal spasm; high-resolution esophageal manometry shows hypertensive peristalsis (first wave on the left) and simultaneous contractions of the esophageal body (second and third wave).

THE LOWER ESOPHAGEAL SPHINCTER

At the distal end of the esophagus lies the LES, located at the gastroesophageal junction. In normal conditions, the LES allows passage of food into the stomach while controlling reflux of gastric contents back into esophagus. Functionally, the LES is best described as two distinct components: the intrinsic and extrinstic sphincters.

At rest, the intrinsic sphincter of the LES is normally comprised of a 2 to 4 cm of tonically contracted smooth muscle dependent on intrinsic myogenic activity [9, 10]. Gross inspection of the LES shows that it is comprised of a thickening of the inner circular muscle layers, which can also be identified through ultrasonography [40, 41]. The resting contractile state of the LES is influenced during fasting in a fashion similar to the stomach and small bowel. Motilin, likely functioning through preganglionic stimulation of cholinergic nerves, establishes synchrony with phases II and III of the migratory motor complex [13-15]. By manometry, normal LES resting pressures are typically 15 to 24 mmHg [27]. During deglutition, the LES relaxes within two seconds of swallowing and stays relaxed for 5 to 10 seconds, corresponding to a cessation of electrical spike activity [11]. After a subsequent 7 to 10 second period of aftercontraction, the LES then resumes its normal resting state (**Fig. 1**). LES relaxation is extremely sensitive and may occur even in the absence of esophageal contraction as occurs during primary or secondary peristalsis [9]. Proper relaxation of the LES is determined by the balance of acetylcholine and substance P (which are excitatory), and non-adrenergic, non-cholinergic neurotransmitters such as NO and VIP (which are inhibitory) [9, 28, 29].

Coordination of LES relaxation and resumption of normal resting pressure has crucial implications in the process of disease. In achalasia, the inhibitory response is lost, resulting in an LES that may or may not be hypertensive, but nonetheless incompletely or partially opens during swallowing (**Fig. 4**) [25]. Pseudoachalasia mimics true achalasia clinically, radiographically, and manometrically (**Fig 5**) [42]. Accounting for 2.4% to 4% of those with possible achalasia, pseudoachalasia is most commonly associated with neoplastic disease, whether arising most commonly from adenocarcinoma at the gastroesophageal junction or more rarely from a metastatic process [43].

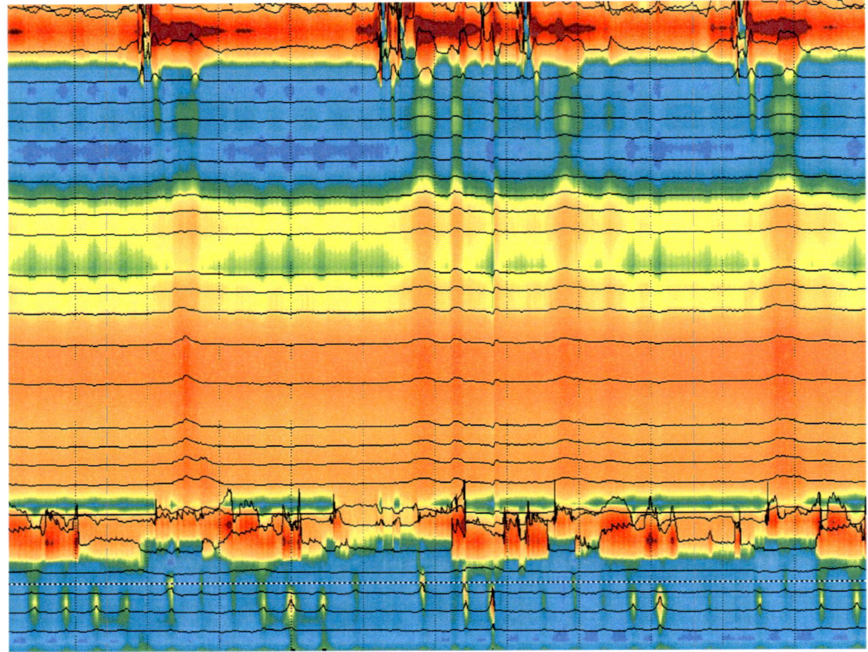

Figure 5. Pseudoachalasia; high-resolution esophageal manometry shows a normotensive LES that rarely relaxes after swallowing. Peristalsis is absent. The patient had a T2N1 adenocarcinoma of the gastroesophageal junction.

Transient LES relaxations, which are independent from swallowing, may account for small amounts of physiologic reflux [31]. However, inappropriate relaxations of the LES may have pathologic implications in reflux disease when they become more frequent or prolonged [12]. Such relaxations have poorly understood causative factors, though post-prandial gastric distention plays a role, and diet and lifestyle (such as cigarette smoking) are implicated as well [4, 16-18]. Further, a hypotensive and/or shortened LES may contribute to reflux disease in many instances. Last, as proposed by DeMeester et al, intraluminal pressure gradients may overcome distal sphincter pressures, and normal activities such as lifting, coughing, or straining, may increase intra-abdominal pressures and account for pathologic reflux seen even in the upright position [34]. Irrespective of the underlying means of sphincter dysfunction, those with reflux-related disease may derive great benefit from surgical correction of reflux. In a study of 300 patients who underwent laparoscopic fundoplication, at one year 91% had normal 24-hour pH studies, 93% absence of heartburn, and 97% overall patient satisfaction [33]. This success of antireflux surgery stems from an increase in the length and resting pressure of the LES, while at the same time in limiting the number and total time of transient relaxation events [31].

Unlike the intrinsic sphincter of the LES, whose tonicity is controlled by smooth muscle, pressures exuded by the extrinsic sphincter of the LES derive mostly from the right crus of the diaphragm [31]. Esophageal manometry reveals oscillations in LES pressures during respiration, with increases of 10 to 20 mmHg during shallow inspiration to 50 to 100 mmHg during deep inspiration [31]. These pressure oscillations have also been noted to correspond proportionally with diaphragmatic contractions as measured by electromyography [19, 20]. As described in the 1950's, the pinchcock action exuded by the extrinsic sphincter is functionally important as it establishes an added level of protection from gastric reflux at periods of increased intra-abdominal pressure as may be seen with coughing or movement [21]. Ultimately, the best example of the extrinsic sphincter's importance is revealed in those with a hiatal hernia, whereby the gastroesophageal junction is displaced superiorly above the diaphragm. Esophageal manometric analysis of the hiatal hernia will demonstrate two independent high pressure zones [4]. The first, cephalad, is created by the resting pressure of the intrinsic component of the LES, and the second, caudad, reflects the pressure created by the right crus of the diaphragm, which now instead of acting on the esophagus, is acting on the herniated gastric wall. This has functional consequences in relation to reflux, as it has been shown that the LES becomes shorter and weaker when larger hiatal hernias are present. This is often accompanied by a worsened degree of esophagitis, reflective of enhanced esophageal acid exposure, diminished acid clearance, and mucosal injury [32].

REFERENCES

[1]   Goyal RK, Martin SB, Shapiro J, Spechler SJ. The role of cricopharyngeus muscle in pharyngoesophageal disorders. *Dysphagia.* 1993;8(3):252-8.

[2]   Sivarao DV, Goyal RK. Functional anatomy and physiology of the upper esophageal sphincter. *Am J Med.* 2000 Mar 6;108 Suppl 4a:27S-37S.

[3] Hammond CS, Davenport PW, Hutchison A, Otto RA. Motor innervation of the cricopharyngeus muscle by the recurrent laryngeal nerve. *J Appl Physiol.* 1997 Jul;83(1):89-94.

[4] Castell DO: Anatomy and physiology of the esophagus and its sphincters. In Castell DO, Diederich LL, Castell JA (eds): *Esophageal Motility and pH Testing.* Colorado, Sandhill Scientific, Inc., 2000, pp 13-28.

[5] Asoh R, Goyal RK. Manometry and electromyography of the upper esophageal sphincter in the opossum. *Gastroenterology.* 1978 Mar;74(3):514-20.

[6] Freiman JM, El-Sharkawy TY, Diamant NE. Effect of bilateral vagosympathetic nerve blockade on response of the dog upper esophageal sphincter (UES) to intraesophageal distention and acid. *Gastroenterology.* 1981 Jul;81(1):78-84.

[7] Gerhardt DC, Shuck TJ, Bordeaux RA, Winship DH. Human upper esophageal sphincter. Response to volume, osmotic, and acid stimuli. *Gastroenterology.* 1978 Aug;75(2):268-74.

[8] Vakil NB, Kahrilas PJ, Dodds WJ, Vanagunas A. Absence of an upper esophageal sphincter response to acid reflux. *Am J Gastroenterol.* 1989 Jun;84(6):606-10.

[9] Goyal RK, Prasad M, Chang HY. *Functional anatomy and physiology of swallowing and esophageal motility.* In: Castell DO, Richter JE. The Esophagus, 4th Edition. Philadelphia, Lippincott Williams & Wilkins, 2004, 1-36.

[10] Goyal RK, Rattan S. Genesis of basal sphincter pressure: effect of tetrodotoxin on lower esophageal sphincter pressure in opossum in vivo. *Gastroenterology.* 1976 Jul;71(1):62-7.

[11] Asoh R, Goyal RK. Electrical activity of the opossum lower esophageal sphincter in vivo. Its role in the basal sphincter pressure. *Gastroenterology.* 1978 May;74(5 Pt 1):835-40.

[12] Dent J, Dodds WJ, Friedman RH, Sekiguchi T, Hogan WJ, Arndorfer RC, Petrie DJ. Mechanism of gastroesophageal reflux in recumbent asymptomatic human subjects. *J Clin Invest.* 1980 Feb;65(2):256-67.

[13] Holloway RH, Blank E, Takahashi I, Dodds WJ, Layman RD. Motilin: a mechanism incorporating the opossum lower esophageal sphincter into the migrating motor complex. *Gastroenterology.* 1985 Sep;89(3):507-15.

[14] Holloway RH, Blank E, Takahashi I, Dodds WJ, Hogan WJ, Dent J. Variability of lower esophageal sphincter pressure in the fasted unanesthetized opossum. *Am J Physiol.* 1985 Apr;248(4 Pt 1):G398-406.

[15] Dent J, Dodds WJ, Sekiguchi T, Hogan WJ, Arndorfer RC. Interdigestive phasic contractions of the human lower esophageal sphincter. *Gastroenterology.* 1983 Mar;84(3):453-60.

[16] Holloway RH, Hongo M, Berger K, McCallum RW. Gastric distention: a mechanism for postprandial gastroesophageal reflux. *Gastroenterology.* 1985 Oct;89(4):779-84.

[17] Wright LE, Castell DO. The adverse effect of chocolate on lower esophageal sphincter pressure. *Am J Dig Dis.* 1975 Aug;20(8):703-7.

[18] Kahrilas PJ. Cigarette smoking and gastroesophageal reflux disease. *Dig Dis.* 1992;10(2):61-71. Review.

[19] Mittal RK, Rochester DF, McCallum RW. Electrical and mechanical activity in the human lower esophageal sphincter during diaphragmatic contraction. *J Clin Invest.* 1988 Apr;81(4):1182-9.

[20] Boyle JT, Altschuler SM, Nixon TE, Tuchman DN, Pack AI, Cohen S. Role of the diaphragm in the genesis of lower esophageal sphincter pressure in the cat. *Gastroenterology.* 1985 Mar;88(3):723-30.

[21] Ingelfinger FJ. Esophageal motility. *Physiol Rev.* 1958 Oct;38(4):533-84.

[22] Kahrilas PJ, Dodds WJ, Hogan WJ. Effect of peristaltic dysfunction on esophageal volume clearance. *Gastroenterology.* 1988 Jan;94(1):73-80.

[23] Leite LP, Johnston BT, Barrett J, Castell JA, Castell DO. Ineffective esophageal motility (IEM): the primary finding in patients with nonspecific esophageal motility disorder. *Dig Dis Sci.* 1997 Sep;42(9):1859-65.

[24] Fouad YM, Katz PO, Hatlebakk JG, Castell DO. Ineffective esophageal motility: the most common motility abnormality in patients with GERD-associated respiratory symptoms. *Am J Gastroenterol.* 1999 Jun;94(6):1464-7.

[25] Fisichella PM, Raz D, Palazzo F, Niponmick I, Patti MG. Clinical, radiological, and manometric profile in 145 patients with untreated achalasia. *World J Surg.* 2008 Sep;32(9):1974-9.

[26] Spechler SJ, Castell DO. *Nonachalasia esophageal motility abnormalities*. In: Castell DO, Richter JE. The Esophagus, 4th Edition. Philadelphia, Lippincott Williams & Wilkins, 2004, 262-74.

[27] Stein HJ, Liebermann-Meffert D, DeMeester TR, Siewert JR. Three-dimensional pressure image and muscular structure of the human lower esophageal sphincter. *Surgery*. 1995 Jun;117(6):692-8.

[28] Dodds WJ, Dent J, Hogan WJ, Arndorfer RC. Effect of atropine on esophageal motor function in humans. *Am J Physiol*. 1981 Apr;240(4):G290-6.

[29] Aggestrup S, Uddman R, Jensen SL, Håkanson R, Sundler F, Schaffalitzky de Muckadell O, Emson P. Regulatory peptides in lower esophageal sphincter of pig and man. *Dig Dis Sci*. 1986 Dec;31(12):1370-5.

[30] Ireland AC, Holloway RH, Toouli J, Dent J. Mechanisms underlying the antireflux action of fundoplication. *Gut*. 1993 Mar;34(3):303-8.

[31] Patti MG, Cantert W, Way LW. Surgery of the esophagus. Anatomy and physiology. *Surg. Clin. North Am*. 1997;77:959-70.

[32] Patti MG, Goldberg HI, Arcerito M, Bortolasi L, Tong J, Way LW. Hiatal hernia size affects lower esophageal sphincter function, esophageal acid exposure, and the degree of mucosal injury. *Am J Surg*. 1996 Jan;171(1):182-6.

[33] Hunter JG, Trus TL, Branum GD, Waring JP, Wood WC. A physiologic approach to laparoscopic fundoplication for gastroesophageal reflux disease. *Ann Surg*. 1996 Jun;223(6):673-85; discussion 685-7.

[34] Demeester TR, Johnson LF, Joseph GJ, Toscano MS, Hall AW, Skinner DB. Patterns of gastroesophageal reflux in health and disease. *Ann Surg*. 1976 Oct;184(4):459-70.

[35] Pearl KP: Anatomy of the esophagus and posterior mediastinum. In Nyhus LM, Baker RJ (eds): *Mastery of Surgery*. Boston, Little, Brown & Company, 1992.

[36] Castell DO: Anatomy and physiology of the esophagus and its sphincters. In Castell DO, Richter JE, Boag Dalton C (eds): *Esophageal Motility Testing*. New York, Elsevier Science, 1987, pp 13-27.

[37] Pellegrini CA, Way LW*: Esophagus and diaphragm*. In Way LW (ed): Current Surgical Diagnosis and Treatment. Stamford, CT, Appleton & Lange, 1994.

[38] Bonington A, Mahon M, Whitmore I. A histological and histochemical study of the cricopharyngeus muscle in man. *J Anat.* 1988 Feb;156:27-37.

[39] Bonington A, Whitmore I, Mahon M. A histological and histochemical study of the cricopharyngeus muscle in the guinea-pig. *J Anat.* 1987 Aug;153:151-61.

[40] Paterson WG, Zhang Y. The lower esophageal sphincter. *Clin Invest Med.* 2002 Feb-Apr;25(1-2):47-53.

[41] Liu JB, Miller LS, Goldberg BB, Feld RI, Alexander AA, Needleman L, Castell DO, Klenn PJ, Millward CL. Transnasal US of the esophagus: preliminary morphologic and function studies. *Radiology.* 1992 Sep;184(3):721-7.

[42] Seo P. Cases from the Osler Medical Service at Johns Hopkins University. Pseudoachalasia due to esophageal adenocarcinoma. *Am J Med.* 2002 Oct 15;113(6):522-4.

[43] Liu W, Fackler W, Rice TW, Richter JE, Achkar E, Goldblum JR. The pathogenesis of pseudoachalasia: a clinicopathologic study of 13 cases of a rare entity. *Am J Surg Pathol.* 2002 Jun;26(6):784-8.

In: Reflux Disease: Causes, Symptoms and ...   ISBN: 978-1-61668-694-9
Editor: G. M. Esposito, pp. 157-171   © 2010 Nova Science Publishers, Inc.

Chapter VII

Obstructive Sleep Apnoea Syndrome and Gastroesophageal Reflux Disease

E. Esteller, I. Modolell and F. Segarra*

Capio Hospital General de Cataluña, San Cugat del Vallès, Barcelona,
Spain.

Gastroesophageal Reflux Disease (GERD) is a very common pathology in the general population and has been connected to various disorders of the respiratory tract [1-3] for some time. At the otorhinolaryngological level, it has been considered a causal or favouring factor of chronic cough, laryngitis, sinusitis, laryngeal stenosis, and carcinoma of the larynx as well as respiratory trouble during sleep [1,3-7].

The exact incidence of gastroesophageal reflux is not known, although it is believed that at least 25% of patients with acid reflux have symptoms at the upper aerodigestive tract:

Dysphonia, postnasal drip, vocal changes, persistent cough, hysterical globus, otalgia, need to constanty clear the throat, halitosis and sleep apnoea.

---

* Correspondence concerning this article should be addressed to: E. Esteller, Hospital General de Catalunya, Calle Pere i Pons, 08190 Sant Cugat del Vallès, Barcelona, Spain. E-mail address: esteller@abaforum.es

[8,9]. It is estimated that between 4 and 10% of consultations in the otorhinolaryngology department are for symptoms related to GERD [2,3,8]. Nevertheless, endoscopic esophagitis is only found in less than 25% of those patients [10]. In addition, a significant percentage of patients with upper aerodigestive tract complaints and GERD do not present typical acid reflux symptoms (burning, indigestion). According to Toohill, this percentage is around 20% [2].

Many patients initially deny clinical symptoms, such as heartburn or regurgitation, but once treated with antacids refer an improvement in symptoms that they had not previously connected with acid reflux [8,2]. Thus, anti-reflux treatment has frequently been used to test the disappearance of upper aerodigestive tract trouble. This last factor seems to be the best diagnostic indicator and the best evidence that reflux is a cause of the symptoms [2].

GERD effect on the pathology of the upper aerodigestive tract may be a direct result of acid reflux, affecting the mucociliar flow, for example, or may be due to a vagal reflex stimulation that causes cough and sore throat and, as a consequence, lesions and symptoms in the area. The extension of this negative effect on the mucosa of the upper aerodigestive tract is proportional to the amount of time of acid exposure and its intensity. Other basic patient problems should be considered as well (vocal abuse, cigarette use, or associated illnesses) [8,11].

It is also known that small amounts of acid are capable of altering the upper aerodigestive tract. This is probably secondary to the tract not being continuously protected by saliva, so the acid reflux can not be mechanically neutralised, favouring the development of lesions. Another probable cause is that, as the mucous is not habitually exposed to these acid levels, the intrinsic cellular mechanisms to protect against chemical injury are not present [11].

Obstructive sleep apnoea syndrome (OSA) and extraesophageal reflux are common chronic illnesses and share several risk factors. The prevalence of acid reflux in OSA patients is significantly higher than in the general population, although casual or temporal relationships have not been yet demonstrated between the two processes [12].

It has not been possible to demonstrate whether a causal relationship really exists between sleep disturbances and proximal acid reflux episodes, or if what actually happens is that the presence of common risk factors frequently leads to both pathologies in the same individual [13-15].

It is well known that a majority of patients with GERD, complain of nocturnal symptoms [16,17]. Nocturnal gastroesophageal reflux is common in individuals with respiratory disturbances such as asthma or OSA, and can affect the severity and frequency of these respiratory disturbances [17]. We also know that, especially at night, gastroesophageal reflux is characterised by a prolonged esophageal acid exposure [16].

Nocturnal gastroesophageal reflux is a common complaint and can disturb sleep: increasing the presence of microarousals and broken sleep [18]. In 2004, Guda, with questionnaires on gastroesophageal reflux symptoms and through nocturnal Polysomnography (PSG), showed that the patients with reflux symptoms have a significantly greater frequency of microarousals, less Phase II sleep and worse tests of quality of life regarding aspects related to aspects of sleep [18].

In 2000, Ing carried out a controlled study where monitored night time pH results were compared in patients with OSA with an apnoea-hypopnea index (AHI) lower than 5 and with a group with AHI higher than 15. In the cases where AHI was higher than 15, a greater number of reflux episodes was observed and the pH measurements were less than 4 for a significant proportion of time compared with the group with AHI lower than 5 (21.4 vs. 3.7%). The majority of acid reflux episodes were related to the amount of time with apnoeas and hypopneas [19]. A possible explanation for this could be that the increase in negative intrathoracic and transdiaphragmatic pressure facilitates acid reflux episodes during the episodes of apnoea [5].

Gastroesophageal reflux (GER) is a phenomenon in that the determinant or fundamental factor is the incompetence of the lower oesophageal sphincter (LES). Thus, a deficient LES would bring about a retrograde flow of gastric contents in the presence of an increase in the pressure gradient between the abdominal and thoracic cavities. Given the extreme negative pressures created by obstruction in patients with OSA, it would be reasonable to assume that this population is at risk for nocturnal gastroesophageal reflux [1,6,20].

In a study on animals designed to determine if the gastroesophageal reflux is related or not to changes in negative inspiratory pressure, Boesch concluded that the changes in said pressure and the gastroesophageal reflux indexes are significantly connected in a positive way. That is, the severity of RGE is correlated with changes in negative inspiratory pressure [21].

On the other hand, RGE can contribute to the appearance of night time apnoeas. Anomalies can occur in the pharyngeal or laryngeal neuromuscular activity as a direct effect of gastric juice above the laryngopharyngeal tissues or through neural activity mediated by reflexes on the larynx and pharynx similar to those observed in the lung when a reflex bronchospasm occurs in the presence of gastroesophageal reflux [5,20].

Finally, this increased risk can be associated with a slowdown in the clearance of acid during the night due to the suppression of normal esophageal clearing mechanisms: salivation and esophageal peristaltism [20,22]. It has been demonstrated that proximal migration of acid in the distal esophagus often occurs during sleep [20].

In Ing's study with PSG on a group of patients with GERD and a control group to see the simultaneous occurrence of obstructive events and acid reflux, it was found that patients with OSA had significantly pH elevations more often than those in the control group. However, only a little more than half of the reflux episodes were related in time to those with apnoea or hypopnea. Subsequently, it was found that the treatment with nasal continuous positive airway pressure (nCPAP) reduced the episodes of reflux in both groups. The authors conclude that gastroesophageal reflux does not appear to be caused by OSA, but can be involved in the pathogenesis of microarousals [19]. This last point is particularly important as certain laboratory studies have suggested that microarousals play a role in the clearance of acid in the distal esophagus during sleep [23].

Some studies find a causal relationship between both pathologies and some authors demonstrate that many night time acid reflux episodes coincide in time with apnoeas and hypopneas [19]. Nevertheless, others, in spite of agreeing with the coincidence of both disorders, do not find a direct relationship [13,24].

A recent project by Kim in 2005 in a Sleep Unit was based on carrying out an investigation with a questionnaire on gastroesophageal reflux symptoms among 1023 patients with OSA diagnosed via PSG. This author found no relationship between OSA and symptoms of gastroesophageal reflux, nor between the severity of OSA and the probability of presenting symptoms of gastroesophageal reflux [25].

In 2004, Berg investigated if the acidification of the distal esophagus that occurs during sleep in subjects with suspected OSA was related to respiratory anomalies. Fourteen males with excessive daytime sleepiness and suspected of having OSA, underwent a PSG, measuring esophageal pressure and pH. It was found that 81% of the reductions in pH lower or equal to 1 were associated with respiratory disturbances. In spite of this, no relationship was found between pH drop and the amount of esophageal pressure, nor with AHI. They concluded that the episodes of esophageal acidification are common in patients with OSA and usually are associated with respiratory events and changes in esophageal pressure. Nevertheless, in the study, pH changes turned out to be independent of the level of esophageal pressure [26].

The opinion of the authors, who do not accept a correlation, is that there are disturbances or common risk factors for both illnesses that cause them to coincide. In fact, characteristic traits of OSA such as obesity and alcohol are also risk factors for GERD [14,15,24,27]. As Orr showed, it is difficult to establish a causal relationship between phenomena that occur with a high level of frequency in the general population and call for a sophisticated statistic analysis. Thus, snoring and burning are very common and it would be expected that both appear associated in any randomly selected population [23].

Nevertheless, there are arguments against authors who deny a direct relationship. In reference to obesity, Gislasson has shown that GER is a risk factor of OSA independent of body mass index (BMI) [5]. These findings were corroborated by Kjelin, who showed that GER in obese patients does not always reduce with weight loss [28].

The methodology of these projects was also criticised. The studies, which denied this relationship, as did those of Penzel and Valipour, used clinical questionnaires to assess the presence of gastroesophageal reflux, when it is fully accepted that the symptoms of reflux are often negative in spite of positive pH measurements [1,29,30].

The study conducted by Graf concluded that no evident relationship exists between respiratory obstructive episodes and reflux episodes. Nevertheless, the assessment of OSA was carried out only with the assessment of a decline in the saturation of O2 of approximately 4% and this cut off probably omitted moderate obstructive episodes that could have altered the conclusions [1,13].

We consider that OSA and GERD are two pathologies that appear to coexist in a significant number of cases, whether through causal relationship of one to the other, through shared risk factors or, very probably, because one aggravates the other.

We are carrying out a prospective study on the effectiveness of treatment with proton pump inhibitors (PPIs) in cases of light or moderate OSA [31]. The preliminary analysis on the time-related relationship, both proximal and distal, of the episodes of pH decline and the respiratory events (analysing apnoeas, hypoapnoeas, desaturations, arousals and waking) show no significant time-related relationship. Nevertheless, we consider it important that a high percentage of our patients with OSA symptoms present significant amounts of proximal and distal reflux determined from 24 hour double canal pH readings, making PPI therapy a coherent alternative that is worth analysis.

Another prospective relationship between both pathologies has been established observing the therapeutic effects of one on the other. Some achieved significant reductions in AHI with medical anti-reflux treatment [32,33]. Others, in contrast, consider that the GER treatment can not reduce the severity of OSA and that it does improve the level of microarousals [19,34].

On the other hand, some projects have managed to demonstrate a cross benefit of specific treatments. Thus, some patients with moderate sleep apnoea symptoms have benefited from treatment with PPI [32,33]. It has also been possible to show a reduction in reflux in patients with or without OSA, through treatment with nCPAP [4].

The treatment with nCPAP seems to achieve a reduction in the intensity of GER both in patients with and without OSA [12,19,35]. Other authors have shown that use of nCPAP in some patients with OSA reduces the symptoms and intensity of GER [4,12,36], including patients who do not respond to treatment with PPI [37]. Nevertheless, the improvement in night time reflux may not be related directly to the effect of continued positive pressure on OSA; since, as intraesophageal pressure and LES pressure increases, it can reduce reflux even in patients without OSA [35].

In daily practice, we meet many patients with light or moderate OSA in whom the application of nCPAP seem disproportionate to their symptoms, patients who do not present anatomical disturbances which justify surgery or which rejected surgical intervention. In this group of patients, we have to try other therapeutical alternatives.

Therapeutic proposals for surgery or nCPAP are usually reluctantly accepted by patients, especially those with moderate or light cases and with limited daytime symptoms. In our opinion, it is necessary to find alternatives to nCPAP and surgery in patients with OSA, especially in non-serious cases, which are the most common. If surgery is not an option for the patient, and he does not have AHI levels to warrant nCPAP or he rejects it, we cannot leave it to chance or tell him that his only option is to lose weight.

When seeking other alternatives, the response of patients is very positive.

These alternative treatments can work in isolation or jointly with others, or even interspersed over time, and the results can be sufficient in many cases. It is important to have a full therapeutic arsenal suitable for providing the best solution for each case, that is, to permit individualizations of the treatment.

Currently, we can consider mandibular advancement devices or postural treatment as well as alternative pharmacological therapy.

As regards the search for a potential pharmacological treatment for OSA, more than 100 drugs for the treatment of OSA have been used with limited results. In general, studies were performed in small series and were often not controlled, and we know practically nothing about their long-term effects [38,39].

In general, these drugs seek to or actually do reduce the REM phase (where the majority of apnoeas occur), increasing the air flow or the muscular tone of dilators during sleep [40].

Clonidine has been tested with the aim of reducing REM Various antidepressants have also been used to reduce the REM phase and preferentially activate the muscles of the dilatory air tract. Acetazolamide, teofiline, nicotine, opiate antagonists and medroxyprogesteronehan have been used to increase ventilation. Acetazolamide appears to reduce central apnoeas in selected patients. However, it is not a drug which is well tolerated and there is not a significant symptomatic response [38-40].

In recent years, the role of selective inhibitors of serotonin recapture has been investigated. An example of this is mirtazapine which increases the activity of the genioglossus, thus widewing the oropharynx [41]. Therefore, the pharmacologic investigation in OSA could be focused in this group of substances, as well as in the pharmacological control of the motor neurons that regulate the upper airway.

On the other hand, given the important role of inflammatory mechanisms in complications related to OSA, it would be theoretically possible that drugs, such as aspirin and statins, which have been shown to be capable of reduce inflammatory components, could have a beneficial or protective effect in patients with OSA [38,39].

The nose plays a disputed role in the physiopathology of OSA. It is now considered that nasal obstruction is a contributing factor in the development of OSA, so resolving it, achieves an improvement in airway passage but not cure OSA [42,43].

Various studies have pointed to the possibility of treating chronic roncopathy and moderate sleep apnoea using topical nasal drugs in patients with nasal obstruction regardless of the presence of allergic rhinitis. There is a high level of agreement that such treatment does not significantly reduce the objective levels of AHI in the vast majority of cases, but it can improve the quality of night time sleep, broken sleep and in some cases, tolerance and compliance of CPAP treatment [42,43].

Medical treatment of nasal pathology should be included in the therapeutic arsenal for light OSA and snoring and as a complement to other treatments in more serious OSA cases. This treatment can improve physical tolerance of CPAP or even reduce the intensity of necessary pressure. Therefore, it may allow titration of CPAP pressure [44].

Nowadays, anti-reflux treatment with PPIs should be considered in these patients. In our opinion, the key issue in this is not so much to show or deny a causal relationship between GERD and OSA, but to try to increase the therapeutic arsenal for OSA with a less aggressive and more comfortable treatment.

Earlier, we explained on the relationship between respiratory pathologies, such as asthma or OSA, and the presence of night time reflux. In these cases the treatment of choice for night time GERD symptoms are PPI. These drugs, which exhibit a rapid and prolonged control of acid secretion, can be particularly useful in treating the night time symptoms of GERD [17].

In 2005, Bortolotti published his results of whether treatment with Omeprazole reduces episodes of night sleep apnoea. He studied 20 OSA patients with a positive PSG and a positive esophageal pHmetry. He asked these patients to keep a diary of apnoea attacks over a four week period. They were treated with either 20 mg omperazole or placebo for six weeks. The average episodes of apnoea per week were significantly reduced in the omeprazole group. This reduction was significant from the third week, reaching a reduction of 73% in the sixth week. Acid reflux may play a role in triggering or aggravating OSA [45].

In 2005, Johnson examined the effects of esomeprazole on night time heartburn, GERD-related sleep disturbances, sleep quality, working productivity and regular activities. It was a multi-centric, randomised, double/blind study in adults with GER-related sleep disturbances and moderate to severe night time heartburn (as registered by the patient's diary). The patients received esomeprazole 40 mg (220 cases), 20 mg (226 cases) or placebo (229 cases) for four weeks. Night time heartburn was reduced 53.1% (111/209) in the first group, 50.5% (111/220) in the second and 12.7% (28/221) in the placebo group. The differences with the placebo group were highly significant. GERD-related sleep disturbances were also significant (73.7% or 73.2% versus 41.2% in the placebo group). Esomeprazole also improved quality of sleep (higher scores on the Pittsburgh Sleep Quality Index (PSQI) (p<0.0001) and saved more work hours per week, according to the Work Productivity and Activity Impairment questionnaire.

Our experience in treating patients with PPIs with mild or moderate OSA (AHI lower than 40) is positive. In 2005, we published a preliminary study where we described the design of the study [31]: all patients who came for a consultation with symptoms suggesting OSA, were offered the opportunity to participate in our study.

The habitual anamnesis of these patients focused on breathing disturbances in sleep (including the Epworth Scale for sleepiness). They were, also, questioned on typical and atypical symptoms of gastroesophageal reflux. Physical examination of these patients included rhinoscopy, oropharyngoscopy, indirect laryngoscopy and flexible endoscopy. We noted the presence of lesions related to reflux: erythema or edema of posterior hemilarynx, presence of granulomas, vocal nodules, or laryngeal scar lesions. Subsequently, we performed conventional polysomnographic study with a 24 hour two-channel pHmetry, so that the polysomnographic readings coincide with the day in which the patient is wearing the bi-channel pH sensor

We consider proximal reflux as significant when the total time pH was ≤4 is equal or over 1% of the total examination time. We evaluated whether the placement of the pHmetry probe would interfere with the PSG results obtained. Data from the polysomnography results of the problem cases were compared with a control group of 55 consecutive cases in those that had a polysomnograph study without pH determination between August and October 2004.

Both populations were comparable in age, sex, BMI and AHI. In both groups, the percentage of effective sleep, the proportions of distinct sleep phases, number of microarousals and awakenings and sleep latency were analysed. None of these variables showed significant differences between the two populations (Table 1).

Table 1. Evaluation of Possible Interference of Phmetry Readings in Sleep Parameters [31]

Parameter	Control Group (55)	Study Group (18)	Statistic
Effective sleep	83.2±10.1	83.6±11.7	NS
Phase 3-4	10.3±6.6	9.8±6.7	NS
REM Phase	15.4±7.3	14.4±6.7	NS
Awakenings	13.3±7.7	9.4±5.9	NS
Arousals	97±89.9	89.4±63.9	NS
Latency	23.8±17.7	29.9±41.8	NS

Carrying out the PSG and pHmetry simultaneously did not show any distortion in the results of our study.

In a speech at the Spanish National Conference in November 2005 in Madrid [46], we showed the first results: From January 2004 until July 2005, 120 patients were included, and a first PSG was performed. Of these, 87 (72.5%) cases had also undergone pHmetry and accepted to join the study. It should be noted that there was a high level of acceptance of undergoing the pHmetry when the patient was explained that we were trying to find an alternative to CPAP or surgery.

Of the 74 cases in which PSG and pHmetry had been done, the latter test had a positive result in the proximal sensor in 34 cases (46%). Of these 34 patients with positive proximal pHmetry, 30 were treated with Pantoprazole, 40 mg daily for at least three months. The four remaining cases had AHI indexes above 40, so we proceeded directly to nCPAP application. The average apnoea-hypoapnoea index of the cases with positive proximal pHmetry treated exclusively with PPI was 15.20±20.6 and average BMI was 27.30±4.3.

Of the 30 treated cases, we obtained a useful follow-up (longer than 3 months) in 20 cases. The results showed an evident clinical improvement in the symptoms of sleep and reflux in 14 (73.7%) and instrumental improvement (PSG) in 8 of the 11 cases in which the control inspection was done (72.7%).

We understand that treatment with PPIs can be a good therapeutic alternative for light or moderate OSA cases. Nevertheless, further investigation is needed as there are still questions to be answered.

One of the key issues is detecting those cases attending our OSA clinic for a consultation, who could be candidates for a double channel 24-hour pHmetry associated with PSG. To date, the initial data from our studies does not enable us to draw conclusions in this area. The symptoms or signs of reflux are not at all demonstrative of whether real reflux exists or not, nor of the eventual therapeutic response.

We must also identify which cases, once studied via PSG and 24-hour pHmetry, have a greater probability of responding to prolonged treatment with PPIs, and whether this treatment is dosage-dependent.

Our current lines of investigation are focused on shining a light on these questions.

REFERENCES

[1] Field SK, Flemons WW. Is the relationship between obstructive sleep apnoea and gastroesophageal reflux clinically important? *Chest* 2002; 121: 1730-1733.

[2] Toohill RJ, Kuhn JC. Role of refluxed acid in pathogenesis of laryngeal disorders. *Am J Med* 1997 Nov 24;103(5A):100S-106S .

[3] Koufman J.A. The otolaryngologic manifestations of gastroesophageal reflux disease (GERD): a clinical investigation of 225 patients using ambulatory 24-hour pH monitoring and an experimental investigation of the role of acid and pepsin in the development of laryngeal injury. *Laryngoscope* 1991; 101 (Suppl 53): 1-78.

[4] Green BT, Broughton WA, O'Connor JB. Marked improvement in nocturnal gastroesophageal reflux in a large cohort of patients with obstructive sleep apnoea treated with continuous positive airway pressure. *Arch Intern Med* 2003;163(1):41-5.

[5] Gislason T, Janson C, Vermeire P, Plaschke P, Bjornsson E, Gislason D, Boman G. Respiratory symptoms and nocturnal gastroesophageal reflux: a population-based study of young adults in three European countries. *Chest.* 2002;121(1):158-63.

[6] Demeter P., Vardi V.K., Magyar P. Study on connection between gastroesophageal reflux disease and obstructive sleep apnoea *Orv Hetil* 2004; 145 (37): 1897-901.

[7] Johnson D.A., Orr W.C., Crawley J.A., Traxler B., McCullough J., Brown K.A., Roth T. Effect of Esomeprazole on Nighttime Heartburn and Sleep Quality in Patients with GERD: A Randomized, Placebo-Controlled Trial. *Am J Gastroenterol* 2005; 100 (9): 1914-1922.

[8] Gaynor EB. Otolaryngologic manifestations of gastroesophageal reflux. *Am J Gastroenterol* 1991 Jul; 86(7):801-8.

[9] Smullen JL, Lejeune FE Jr. Otolaryngologic manifestations of gastroesophageal reflux disease. *J La State Med Soc* 1999 Mar; 151(3):115-9.

[10] Klinkenberg-Knol EC. Otolaryngologic manifestations of gastro-oesophageal reflux disease. *Scand J Gastroenterol Suppl* 1998; 225:24-8.

[11] Wong RK, Hanson DG, Waring PJ, Shaw G. ENT manifestations of gastroesophageal reflux *Am J Gastroenterol* 2000 Aug; 95(8 Suppl):S15-22.

[12] Zanation A.M., Senior B.A. The relationship between extraesophageal reflux (EER) and obstructive sleep apnoea (OSA). *Sleep Med Rev* 2005; Sep 21.

[13] Graf, KI, Karaus, M, Heinemann, S, Korber S, Dorow P, Hampel KE. Gastroesophageal reflux in patients with sleep apnoea syndrome. *J Gastroenterol* 1995; 33: 689-693.

[14] Valipour A., MD; Himender K. Makker, MD; Rebecca Hardy, PhD; Stephen Emegbo, MSc; Tudor Toma, MD and Stephen G. Spiro, MD Symptomatic Gastroesophageal Reflux in Subjects with a Breathing Sleep Disorder* *Chest.* 2002;121:1748-1753.)

[15] Morse C.A., Quan S.F., Mays M.Z., Green C., Stephen G., Fass R. Is there a relationship between obstructive sleep apnoea and gastroesophageal reflux disease? *Clin Gastroenterol Hepatol* 2004; 2 (9): 761-8.

[16] Jaspersen D., Leodolter A. Sleep disorders associated with gastrooesophageal reflux *Dtsch Med Wochenschr* 2005; 130 (48): 2779-2782.

[17] Orr W.C. Therapeutic Options in the Treatment of Nighttime Gastroesophageal Reflux. *Digestión* 2005; 72 (4): 229-238.

[18] Guda N., Partington S., Vakil N. Symptomatic gastro-oesophageal reflux, arousals and sleep quality in patients undergoing polysomnography for possible obstructive sleep apnoea. *Aliment Pharmacol Ther* 2004; 20 (10): 1153-1159.

[19]Ing, AJ, Ngu, MC, Breslin, AB Obstructive sleep apnoea and gastroesophageal reflux. *Am J Med* 2000; Suppl 4a108:120S-125S.

[20]Orr W.C. Sleep-Related Breathing Disorders. Is It All About Apnoea? *Chest.* 2002;121:8-11.

[21]Boesch R.P., Shah P., Vaynblat M., Marcus M., Pagala M., Narwal S., Kazachkov M. Relationship between upper airway obstruction and gastroesophageal reflux in a dog model. *J Invest Surg* 2005; 18 (5): 241-245.

[22]Teramoto, S, Kume, H, Ouchi, Y Nocturnal gastroesophageal reflux: symptom of obstructive sleep apnoea syndrome in association with impaired swallowing. *Chest* 2002; 122: 2266-2267.

[23]Orr, WC, Johnson, LF, Robinson, MG The effect of sleep on swallowing, esophageal peristalsis, and acid clearance. *Gastroenterology* 1984; 86: 814-819.

[24]Penzel, T, Becker, HF, Brandenburg, U, Labunski T, Pankow W, Peter JH. Arousal in patients with gastro-oesophageal reflux and sleep apnoea. *Eur Respir J* 1999; 14:1266-1270.

[25]Kim H.N., Vorona R.D., Winn M.P., Doviak M., Johnson D.A , Catesby W. Symptoms of gastro-oesophageal reflux disease and the severity of obstructive sleep apnoea syndrome are not related in sleep disorders center patients. *Aliment Pharmacol Ther* 2005; 21 (9): 1127-1133.

[26]Berg S, Hoffstein V, Gislason T. Acidification of distal esophagus and sleep-related breathing disturbances. *Chest.* 2004 Jun;125(6):2101-6.

[27]Suganuma N, Shigedo Y, Adachi H, Watanabe T, Kumano-Go T, Terashima K, Mikami A, Sugita Y, Takeda M. Association of gastroesophageal reflux disease with weight gain and apnoea, and their disturbance on sleep. *Psychiatry Clin Neurosci* 2001; 55(3):255-6.

[28]Kjelin A., Ramel, S, Rossner, S, Thor, K Gastroesophageal reflux in obese patients is not reduced by weight reduction. *Scan J Gastroenterol* 1996; 31:1047-1051.

[29]Teramoto S., MD; Hiroshi Yamamoto, MD and Yasuyoshi Ouchi, MD Gastroesophageal Reflux Common in Patients with Sleep Apnoea Rather Than Snorers Without Sleep Apnoea *Chest.* 2003;124:767-768.

[30]Harding, SM, Guzzo, MR, Richter, JE The prevalence of gastroesophageal reflux in asthma patients without reflux symptoms. *Am J Respir Crit Care Med* 2000; 162: 34-39.

[31] E. Esteller, I. Modolell, F. Segarra, E. Matiñó, A. Enrique, JM.Ademà and E. Estivill Reflujo gastroesofágico proximal y síndrome de la apnea obstructiva del sueño. *Acta Otorrinolaringol Esp* 2005; 56 (9):411-415.

[32] Senior, BA, Khan, M, Schwimmer, C, Rosenthal L, Benninger M. Gastroesophageal reflux and obstructive sleep apnoea. *Laryngoscope* 2001; 111: 2144-2146

[33] Xiao G, Wang Z, Ke M, et al. *The relationship between obstructive sleep apnoea and gastroesophageal reflux and the effect of antireflux therapy* Zhonghua Nei Ke Za Zhi. 1999; 38(1):33-6.

[34] Steward DL. Pantoprazole for sleepiness associated with acid reflux and obstructive sleep disordered breathing. *Laryngoscope.* 2004; 114(9):1525-8.

[35] Kerr, P, Shoenut, JP, Steens, RD, Millar T, Micflikier AB, Kryger MH. Nasal continuous positive airway pressure: a new treatment for nocturnal gastroesophageal reflux? *J Clin Gastroenterol* 1993; 17: 276-280.

[36] Okada, S, Ouchi, Y, Teramoto, S Nasal continuous positive airway pressure and weight loss improve swallowing reflex in patients with obstructive sleep apnoea syndrome. *Respiration* 2000; 67: 464-466.

[37] Konermann M, Radu HJ, Teschler H, Rawert B, Heimbucher J, Sanner BM. Interaction of sleep disturbances and gastroesophageal reflux in chronic laryngitis. *Am J Otolaryngol* 2002;23(1):20-6.

[38] Abad V.C., Guilleminault C Pharmacological management of sleep apnoea. *Expert Opin Pharmacother* 2006; 7 (1): 11-23.

[39] Smith I., Lasserson T., Wright J. Drug therapy for obstructive sleep apnoea in adults *Cochrane Database Syst Rev.* 2006; 19 (2): CD003002.

[40] Richard L. Horner The neuropharmacology of upper airway motor control in the awake and asleep states: implications for obstructive sleep apnoea *Respir Res.* 2001; 2 (5): 286–294.

[41] Castillo J.L., Menendez P., Segovia L., Guilleminault C. Effectiveness of mirtazapine in the treatment of sleep apnoea/hypopnea syndrome (SAHS). *Sleep Med* 2004; 5(5): 507-8.

[42] Kiely JL, Nolan P, McNicholas WT. Intranasal corticosteroid therapy for obstructive sleep apnoea in patients with co-existing rhinitis. *Thorax.* 2004 Jan; 59(1):50-5.

[43] Hughes K, Glass C, Ripchinski M, Gurevich F, Weaver TE, Lehman E, Fisher LH, Craig TJ. Efficacy of the topical nasal steroid budesonide on

improving sleep and daytime somnolence in patients with perennial allergic rhinitis *Allergy*. 2003 May; 58(5):380-5.

[44]E. Esteller, E. Matiñó, F. Segarra, J.J. Sanz, J.M. Ademà, E. Estivill: Efectos adversos derivados del tratamiento con nCPAP y su relación con la nariz. *Acta Otorrinolaringol Esp* 2004; 55:17-22.

[45]Bortolotti M., Gentilini L., Morselli C., Giovannini M. Obstructive sleep apnoea is improved by a prolonged treatment of gastrooesophageal reflux with omeprazole. *Dig Liver Dis* 2005; Oct 24.

[46]Esteller E., Modolell I., Segarra F., Matiñó E. Enrique A. y Ademà JM. OSA and gastroesophageal reflux: a therapeutic alternative. *56th National Conference of the Spanish Society of Otorrinolaringology and Cervical/Facial Pathology*. Madrid 12-15 November 2005.

B

C

G

H

I

P

T

W

X

Y